The *Dietitian* Kitchen

Kerri Major

The *Dietitian* KITCHEN®

Nutrition for a Healthy, Strong, & Happy You

MEYER & MEYER SPORT

British Library of Cataloguing in Publication Data
A catalogue record for this book is available from the British Library

The Dietitian Kitchen®
Maidenhead: Meyer & Meyer Sport (UK) Ltd., 2020
ISBN: 978-1-78255-184-3

Aachen, Auckland, Beirut, Dubai, Hägendorf, Hong Kong, Indianapolis, Cairo, Cape Town, Manila, Maidenhead, New Delhi, Singapore, Sydney, Tehran, Vienna

 Member of the World Sport Publishers' Association (WSPA), www.w-s-p-a.org

Printed by Print Consult, GmbH, Munich, Germany

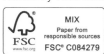

ISBN: 979-1-78255-184-3
Email: info@m-m-sports.com
www.thesportspublisher.com

Contents

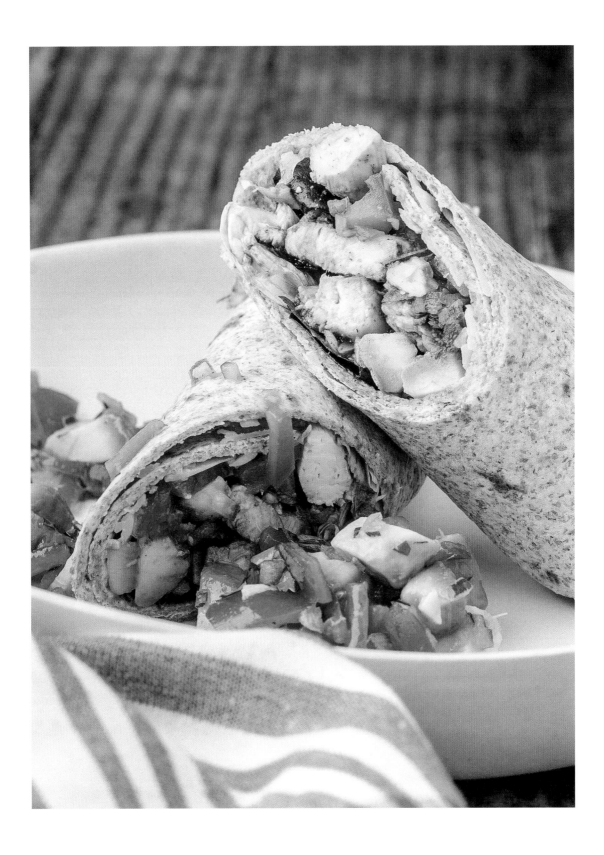

Preface

With a surge in the number of people out there offering 'nutritional advice' and the multi-million-pound diet industry forever growing its prospects, you are probably wondering how this book is going to be any different from all the other food and nutrition books you see out there on the shelves.

This book is a game changer. Many of the food and nutrition books you find on the market today are written by popular celebrities and fitness models, who lack any formal qualifications in health or nutrition. They often promote fad diets and detoxes which are not only bad for your health, but they also fail to provide good quality nutritional advice to help you develop a healthy relationship with food for the long-term.

This book is different. As a qualified Dietitian, Sports Dietitian and Personal Trainer (not to mention a self-confessed foodie who loves to cook – and bake!), I have expertise in both nutrition and exercise. This puts me in the perfect position to provide you with an evidence-based approach to support your all-round health and well-being.

Dietitians are the only nutritional professionals to be regulated by law. We are qualified to assess, diagnose and treat diet- and nutrition-related problems, using the most up-to-date research on food, health and disease. This ensures we always work to the highest standard and that the advice we provide is not only accurate and evidence-based, but also safe. We are trained to translate this information into practical guidance to allow people to make appropriate lifestyle and food choices based on advice they know they can trust.

So, forget the diet. Forget the detox. Forget the quick fix. This book is here to provide you with credible nutrition advice. It features lots of healthy, nourishing and delicious recipes, in addition to fun exercise programmes, to help you fall in love with looking after yourself. This book is about enjoying real food and developing good, sustainable and rewarding health habits. It is about inspiring you to move your body in ways that energise you and make you feel fit and strong. I want to help you appreciate exactly how the food we eat and the way we move have an impact on our overall health and well-being.

My philosophy is simple. I strongly believe nutrition and exercise should be not only simple, but also affordable and enjoyable. I believe that we should be nourishing our bodies with unprocessed, whole foods most of the time, and that we should move our bodies every day in a way that is both fun and empowering, for the mind, body and soul. By doing so, I believe everyone can reach a place where they feel body-confident and where their physical and mental well-being allows them to live life to the absolute fullest.

Enjoy the journey.

Kerri xo

Acknowledgments

First and foremost, I want to say a huge thank you to the team at Meyer and Meyer Sport for giving me this opportunity to write my very own book. Thank you for believing in me and for being so helpful and supportive throughout this whole experience. It has been an absolute honour to work with such a dedicated publisher who shares my passion and enthusiasm for health, nutrition and fitness. I must say a special thank you to Liz, my managing editor, who first saw potential in The Dietitian Kitchen and approached me with this opportunity. You have allowed me to achieve one of my biggest dreams of releasing my own book, and I will be forever grateful. You have been amazing and so unbelievably encouraging and supportive, and it has been a real pleasure working with you. Thank you so much for believing in me.

Thank you to Daniel McAvoy for capturing such beautiful photographs for this book. It has been so much fun working with you and your eye for detail for getting the perfect shot is incredible. You have really helped to bring this book to life and to turn my dreams into reality on the page, in the most beautiful way possible. Thank you for your help and guidance throughout this whole experience.

To the amazing Jack Baxter and Sara Hill, for my beautiful hair and make-up. You kept me looking natural and just like myself in all the photos, through your amazing talent, by keeping me calm, and making me laugh and smile while on set. It was so lovely working with you both.

Thank you to my brilliant friend, Alan Dougan. You are an unbelievable chef and I couldn't have done all of this without your help. Thanks to you, we have been able to capture my recipes so beautifully. I will be forever grateful for your time, guidance, help and support throughout this whole experience.

To the lovely Laurie, a great family friend, for so kindly allowing me to borrow so many of your beautiful plates, dishes and other kitchenware. Your collection of crockery is absolutely stunning, and it has really added something special to the way my recipes were photographed.

To Stephen Fraser, thank you so much for letting me use your beautiful studio, The FITT Principle, to capture some of the fitness photos. Your space is really incredible, and I am so grateful of the opportunity to work with you.

To Maurice Mancini, Gail Barron and Pillow Partners, thank you for letting me use your gorgeous space to capture some beautiful photos. You were so accommodating, and I was so pleased to have found the perfect place right in my own hometown.

Thank you to my amazing Dietitian colleague and friend, Anna Julian for proofreading the book and for all your support and guidance. Your advice was invaluable, and I cannot thank you enough.

To my sister, and best friend, Laura. I am so grateful for all your advice, as well as all the time and patience you have given me throughout this whole experience. Thank you for being my biggest fan and for always being so supportive.

To my Mum and Dad. Where do I begin? I simply cannot put into words just how grateful I am for all you have done for me. You have always believed in me and are always there when I need you. I wouldn't be where I am today if it weren't for you both. You offer so much love and support and you have always given me so much encouragement to help me achieve my dreams. Mum, thank you for helping me develop my passion for cooking. I will never be as good as you, but I will keep trying. Dad, your love and support, not to mention your sense of humour, have always kept me smiling, even during the most difficult and stressful times. Both of you are my rock.

My beautiful Gran, Amy. Thank you for being so supportive and the kindest and most beautiful human on the planet. You created my love for baking from a very young age and it's one of my favourite hobbies, getting in the kitchen with you and making some delicious treats. You are my inspiration.

To the rest of my family and my lovely friends, thank you for being my greatest fans and for always believing in me.

From the bottom of my heart, thank you to my other half, Gary. I thank my lucky stars every day that we found each other. I will be forever grateful for all the love, support and patience that you give to me in everything I do.

Finally, to all of my followers. I wouldn't have had the incredible opportunity to create this book – my dream – if it weren't for you. You inspire and motivate me every day, and I sincerely wish to thank each and every one of you. I really hope you love reading this book, and I hope it brings you great health and happiness.

My Story

Food and fitness have always been a huge part of my life. I have always loved my food and have enjoyed playing sports and keeping active from a young age. Food makes me happy and I am a firm believer that it should make everyone happy. I have been fortunate in that my relationship with food has been relatively 'uncomplicated'. I grew up on my Mum's delicious, hearty meals and her amazing baking, and I have always baked regularly with my lovely Gran. It continues to be a running joke among family and friends, that if I am not my "usual, bubbly self", more often than not, you can just give me some food, and I will be smiling again in no time.

My parents raised me on the importance of everyone sitting down to family meals together, enjoying the food on offer and ensuring that meals were a time where we had limited other distractions and we could enjoy one another's company. I owe it to them for helping me develop my love for food and nutrition, as well as helping me create my own healthy relationship with food.

KEEPING IT REAL

On social media, I have been open about a short period of time in my life where I became quite overly fixated on exactly what I was eating and what my weight showed on the scales. That was the extent of it. I still ate, but I watched exactly what I ate. I restricted 'treats', I ran a lot, and I was more interested in the calories I burned, rather than the actual enjoyment of the exercise I was doing. I weighed myself pretty much daily. I was frustrated and upset when I felt I had eaten "well" but the number on the scales hadn't gone down. My relationship with food and exercise was all wrong, but the fortunate thing for me was, that in my head, I knew this.

It was from taking Home Economics classes in school, that my passion for food and cooking, as well as my curiosity to learn exactly what fueled and nourished my body, started to grow. The more I learned about nutrition, the more my passion for this area grew, and it quickly became clear to me what career path I should be taking. As I began to follow my dream of becoming a Dietitian, my relationship with food, exercise and my body soon repaired itself. I absolutely loved learning about all the nutrients in our food and what their role was in the body. I was fascinated by how the body digests the food we eat and how the food we eat has an impact on our overall health and well-being. I started to really enjoy food again because I knew that what I was eating was good for my health, and I was thriving on it. I started to include 'treat foods' again, enjoying them, just for their sheer deliciousness. I started trying out new forms of exercise, not because I felt I had to, but because I actually wanted to, to help me feel fit and get stronger. And the most rewarding thing of all? I began weighing myself less and less. Why? Because I no longer cared about how much I weighed. I was feeling the best I ever had. I was fueling myself the right way and I was keeping active in ways I actually enjoyed. I was reaping the benefits of increased confidence, better moods and the sheer enjoyment of food and movement again. My relationship with gravity meant nothing to me. It still doesn't. Throwing out my bathroom scales was one of the best things I have ever done.

I come from the generation when social media was born, and I started using all the new social media platforms as they came out. In recent years, it's almost become 'fashionable' to keep a health and wellness social media account, which, unfortunately, has resulted in many people freely offering nutritional advice, when quite frankly, they aren't qualified to do so. I quickly became aware of how much rubbish was being posted on social media with regards to food and exercise, and sadly, this is still the case today. Every day, I see more and more posts on social media advertising fad diets and ridiculous detox programmes. More often than not, these unhealthy trends are being promoted by celebrities or 'social media influencers' who tend to have no qualifications in nutrition, whatsoever. Their large social media following means these products and ideas reach the masses, with many people believing that they must work because these celebrities look great, right? This was the reason I started @The_Dietitian_Kitchen on Instagram and Facebook. I was fed up with the wrong information being put out there on the internet, potentially causing harm to vulnerable individuals and encouraging people to develop a terrible relationship with food, exercise and their bodies. The diet industry is a multi-million-pound business because diets and detoxes generally do NOT work. So people keep looking for the next magic diet that they hope will help them lose weight. This has to stop.

Social media is becoming more and more popular, and for that reason, I believe that Dietitians need to begin to grow their own presence online and bust the nutrition myths that are being spread around the world today. We are the ones with the evidence-based knowledge who can in fact help people.

This is why I feel so unbelievably privileged to be given this opportunity. I am delighted that I can share my nutritional knowledge and expertise with you, in the form of my first-ever book. It has enabled me to gather in one place, all the information and tools that you will need to create a healthy relationship with food. With my knowledge in personal training, I have also provided you with some fun workouts to inspire you to get moving, combining this with my expertise in sports nutrition so that you know exactly how to fuel yourself well for exercise.

I want this book to help inspire you to become healthier, fitter, stronger and happier – and most of all, I want you to love every second of the process. I am really excited to share my vision of food and exercise with you. This book provides you with more than 90 simple, healthy and delicious meal ideas, lots of motivational health and fitness tips, and a bunch of fun workouts to help you become the healthiest, fittest and happiest version of yourself. I also want to help you to develop a healthy and positive relationship with food so you can nourish your body in the right way, ditching the idea that you need to go on a diet or detox to get healthy or lose weight. I honestly believe that no food should be restricted or forbidden, and I hope this book shows you that this is exactly the type of approach that I not only encourage my clients to follow, but which I follow too – the Sweet Indulgence section in this book will not disappoint you! Last, but not least, I want to get rid of the belief that there are certain foods which are 'good' or 'bad', as I believe that every food and drink can have its place in your diet. The key to all of this is not hidden in a diet, a powder, a pill or a so-called 'superfood'. There is no quick fix. It's about improving your knowledge and understanding of nutrition and making enjoyable, sustainable changes that will last a lifetime.

How do I know all this is possible? Because I can speak from personal experience and admit that I am finally in a place where I have a complete balance in my life. It is do-able and the process can be both empowering and rewarding. All you need to do is consider unlearning what you think you already know about nutrition (especially if your main sources of information have been the media and magazines), as well as to have a little bit of self-belief and motivation to get you started. Allow the evidence-based advice in this book to guide, support and inspire you to try new ways of cooking, eating and exercising, leading you on a journey towards better overall health and well-being.

Stay positive, consistent and enthusiastic and just enjoy the journey as you reap the amazing benefits from nourishing your mind, body and soul.

GETTING STARTED

When people learn I am a Dietitian, often the first thing they ask is how exactly can I help them lose weight, usually said with the hope that I will be able to wave a magic wand for them. The majority of people that start this conversation with me have usually tried every quick-fix diet under the sun, and hope that I can provide yet another quick and easy solution for them, to help them drop the pounds. I get it – these quick fixes sound easy, promising and a much simpler way of reaching your goals, but as the saying goes – if something sounds too good to be true, it probably is.

As mentioned before, this is how the diet industry makes its fortune, because far too many people continually look for that quick fix that will work for them long-term, but the truth is, that quick fix doesn't exist. So when one diet doesn't work, another one is tried, and then another, and then another. See where I'm going here? As a result, the diet industry's bank balance just keeps going up and up, and they keep creating more and more fad diets to rob you of your well-earned money.

Fad diets tend to reel people in because people can often achieve immediate weight loss. However, the problems lie when the diet becomes too challenging and too restrictive to maintain long-term, causing people to give up and go back to eating the way they did before. Fad diets usually provide little in the way of any nutrition education. This means people have learned nothing new about how to actually nourish their bodies, often resulting in people regaining all the weight they have just lost, and even more on top of that. And this cycle continues, not only destroying your relationship with food, but also the relationship you have with your body. For this reason, many people don't believe that anything can help them and tend to begin accepting that their struggle with weight loss is just the way life is for them. My promise here is that it really doesn't need to be this way, and the key lies in improving your own nutritional knowledge.

I mentioned earlier – "Enjoy the journey." This is what it is all about. Eating healthy in a way that is good for your mind, body and soul is a journey. It starts with having basic nutritional knowledge so that you know how to fuel yourself the right way. Having a good understanding of the basic nutrition principles will help you to create a healthy and happy relationship to food so you can save money and say goodbye to restrictive fad diets and dodgy diet products.

Taking this first step can seem daunting. There is always a reason for putting something off, particularly when the action itself seems difficult or will bring about a lifestyle change that seems very different to what you're used to. There is never going to be a good time to start, so really there is no better time than now. We are creatures of habit, which means initially, it may be difficult. It may need some dedication and hard work on your part, but remember, changing a lifetime of habits doesn't happen overnight. It's about starting off small, tackling one or two things at a time, and most importantly, being patient with yourself. The nutrition advice and the simple tools and techniques I share in this book, I believe, are essential in providing you with the starting blocks with which to begin your journey. So, all I ask is, that you start with an open mind and a positive attitude, and then simply enjoy your journey towards greater health and feeling on top of the world.

KNOWLEDGE IS POWER

As the saying goes, knowledge is power, and understanding the basics of nutrition is the power that you need in order to eat well for life. Knowing how to eat well has been made unnecessarily difficult for everyone, thanks to so many unqualified people giving out nutrition advice. Without undervaluing my degree (as it was, in no way, shape or form, easy to achieve), the basics of nutrition can, in fact, be relatively simple, and that is what many people have lost sight of.

This is why I want to I encourage you to try and unlearn what you think you already know about nutrition and start all over again. I want to help you understand how to eat a balanced diet so that you can reap the benefits of nourishing your body with amazing food. I want you to view food and exercise in a completely different way, rather than focusing on what impact these can have on your relationship with gravity (i.e. your weight). I want you to say goodbye to the restrictions that often comes with following a diet, while I give you the knowledge and power needed to make your own educated and informed choices about the foods you eat. I want you to see every meal as an opportunity to nourish your body and to know why this is so. That's why you will not find a short-term diet plan in here. I want you to be set up for life, so that you know how to eat well every day. I want to inspire you to find a form of exercise you love because you know and understand why staying active is good for you.

I can't emphasise this enough: The real key to changing how you look and feel must come from a good knowledge and understanding of nutrition and health. This will allow you to make educated and informed choices and can lead you on a path to living a healthy and fulfilling life.

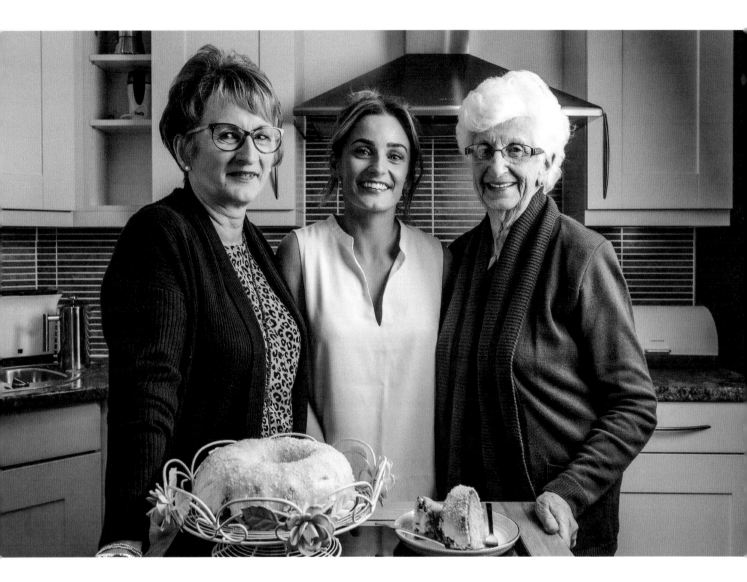

My lovely Mum and Gran, two of the most amazing and inspirational women I know and the two people I have to thank for developing my love for cooking and baking (and not to mention my very sweet tooth!).

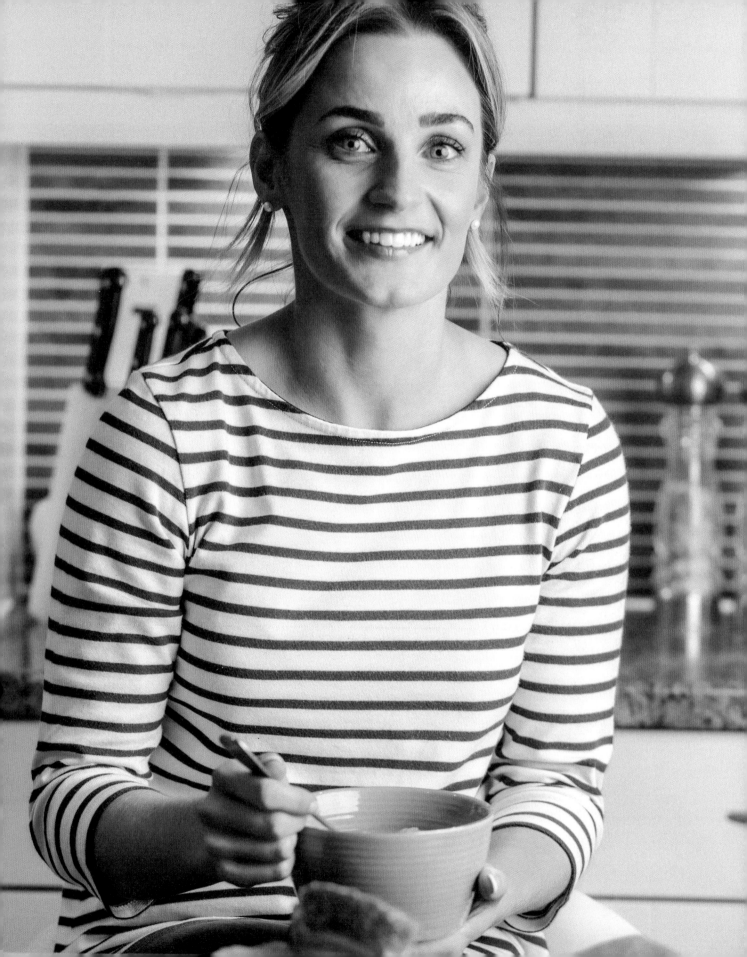

Nutrition

THE BASICS

As mentioned before, this is where I ask you to unlearn everything you have done before with regards to nutrition and read this chapter with a fresh and open mind.

The first thing I always ask people to do, is to consider changing their mindset, believing that how and what we eat should be about so much more than just weight loss. We all need to be thinking about how we can eat better for our health and happiness, rather than how it can help us shed the pounds. Rather than focusing on what we should be cutting out of our diet, our focus should be on what to include, and how we can nourish ourselves with the food we eat.

This can be challenging, and it won't happen overnight. I ask you to be patient and simply enjoy the journey. It's about making a few, small changes at a time and building on this gradually so that you and your body aren't overwhelmed and have enough time to adapt. By concentrating on what should be included in your diet, you will begin to notice that eating well doesn't need to be boring or restrictive. The health improvements you will see, such as increased energy levels, enhanced sleep, improved digestive tract function, better fitting clothes, etc., will only empower you to continue.

Remember: Knowledge is power. Learning and understanding the basic principles of good nutrition is essential to get started and maintain a healthy diet for life. For a diet to be sustainable, it needs to be flexible and enjoyable. This is why you will never find me giving out strict diet plans. Eating healthily should be about eating for pleasure, with no guilt and no restrictions. I would, therefore, much rather encourage you to learn why eating different foods can be good for your health, as well as how you can build a balanced plate yourself so that you have the freedom to make your own appropriate food choices.

This knowledge, flexibility and variety will empower and enable you to eat well for life.

Nutrients

All the food we eat contains nutrients – substances that provide nourishment to the body and which are essential for growth and life. There are five main nutrients in the diet and these can be split into two important groups: Macronutrients and Micronutrients.

Macronutrients are nutrients that are required in large amounts in the diet.

Micronutrients are those that are only required in small amounts.

Macronutrients	Micronutrients
1. Carbohydrates	1. Vitamins
2. Protein	2. Minerals
3. Fat	

MACRONUTRIENTS

All three of the macronutrients provide energy to the body in the form of calories. However, the amount of calories that each macronutrient provides per gram differs.

Macronutrient	Calories (kcal) per gram
1. Carbohydrate	4
2. Protein	4
3. Fat	9

In order to fuel our daily activities, we must give our bodies the energy (calories) they need by providing them with adequate amounts of macronutrients. Looking at the previous table, it is clear that carbohydrates and protein provide the same amount of energy per gram, and fat slightly more. We will touch on calories and energy intake later in the book (see the section, Calories), where I discuss why I strongly encourage you not to count calories but instead to just be calorie conscious. I believe it's important for you to develop an awareness of the energy density of different foods and where exactly the energy in your diet comes from.

In addition to each macronutrient providing you with energy, they also have many other essential functions of their own, so it is important that you include adequate amounts of each macronutrient in your diet every day.

CARBOHYDRATES

Carbohydrates are the main source of energy for the human body, and they can be found in a large variety of different foods. In order for the body to get energy from carbohydrates, the body's digestive system must break down the carbohydrate into its simplest and most basic form, otherwise known as glucose (sugar). Glucose is then transported from the gut into the bloodstream and distributed to all the cells within the body. As it enters each cell, it provides them with energy, allowing them to function. The glucose within the bloodstream is often referred to as 'blood sugar' or 'blood glucose'.

Glucose is the body's preferred source of fuel, especially for the brain, meaning it is really important that we include sources of carbohydrate in our diet on a regular basis.

In order to understand the importance of carbohydrates, we need to consider the different types based on their chemical structures.

1. Complex Carbohydrates
2. Simple (and Free) Carbohydrates

COMPLEX CARBOHYDRATES

Complex carbohydrates, otherwise known as polysaccharides ('poly' meaning 'many'), are carbohydrate foods which are made up of a complex structure of lots of sugar units linked together, (e.g. different combinations of the sugar units known as glucose, fructose, galactose, lactose and sucrose). Complex carbohydrates are often also referred to as 'starchy carbohydrates' and can be found in a large variety of foods, including bread, rice, potatoes, pasta and cereal. Due to their complicated structure, complex carbohydrates are broken down slowly by the body's digestive system to form glucose. It is this slow release of energy which helps keep our bodies well fuelled throughout the day and makes it important for us all to include complex carbohydrates regularly in our diet.

Complex carbohydrates not only provide the body with energy when they are digested, but they can also provide many other nutrients, such as fibre, vitamins and minerals, as well as some protein and healthy fats. We should aim to choose the non-processed, wholegrain forms of complex carbohydrates, (e.g. wholegrain rice, wholegrain pasta, wholegrain bread, etc.) to increase our fibre intake.

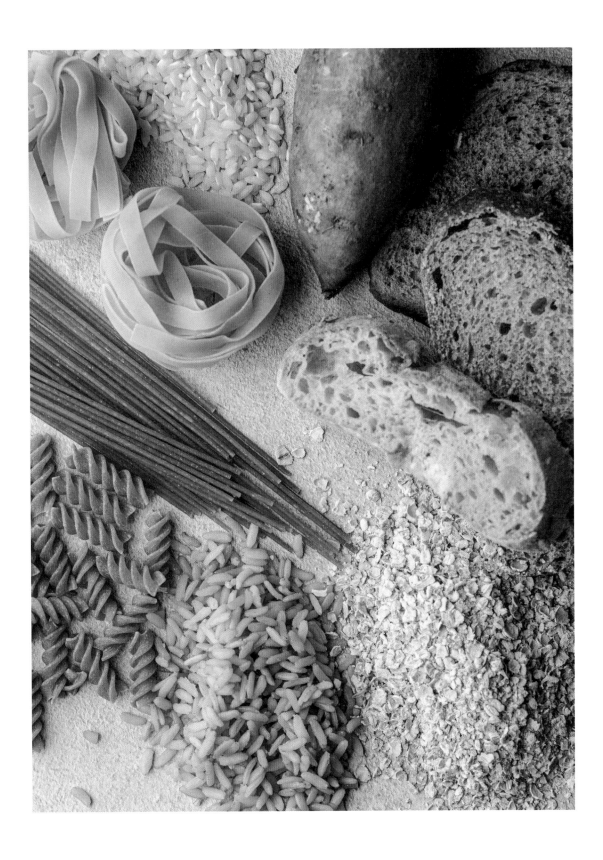

SIMPLE CARBOHYDRATES

Simple carbohydrates, otherwise known as monosaccharides or disaccharides ('mono' meaning one, 'di' meaning 'two'), are carbohydrate foods which are made up of one or two sugar units. This simple structure means they are digested and absorbed quickly and easily by the body and into the bloodstream. They provide us with a quick supply of energy which can be useful at times, especially with regards to fuelling for sport and exercise. This will be covered in more depth in the section, Nutrition for Fitness.

Simple carbohydrates can be found naturally in many foods, such as dairy products, fruit and vegetables, as well as in refined, processed products such as white bread, white rice and white pasta, sweets, biscuits, cakes and sugary drinks. The simple carbohydrates which are found naturally in foods (i.e. dairy products and fruit and vegetables) are important to include regularly in our diet because these are considered nutrient-dense foods, often containing many other nutrients, such as healthy fats, vitamins, minerals and fibre, which are necessary to support our health. However, the refined, processed products often tend to be lacking in many other nutrients so although they provide us with energy, we are recommended to limit our intake of these and enjoy them in moderation.

'Free Sugars' is the term given to any sugars that are added to foods (e.g. sugar added to the refined products mentioned above, i.e. biscuits, chocolate, cakes, sweets, etc.) or sugars which are naturally present in honey, syrups and unsweetened fruit juices. This does not include the sugars found naturally in "whole fruit and vegetables or those found in milk and milk products.

Most of our free sugar intake tends to come from the sugar added to food and drink by manufacturers. Foods containing free sugars often lack in other nutrients, meaning they can easily contribute energy, without contributing more beneficial nutrients. Given that this type of carbohydrate is associated with weight gain and can also contribute to tooth decay, we are recommended to keep our intake of free sugars to a minimum. Guidelines suggest that we all should be limiting our consumption of free sugars to no more than 30g per day (i.e. 7 teaspoons). If you are looking at food labels, when you see the phrase 'of which sugars', this value includes both free and natural sugars and doesn't differentiate between the two. For this reason, it is useful to look at the ingredients list to see the sugars that have been added to the product.

MISLEADING FOOD LABELLING: NATURAL SUGARS VS REFINED SUGARS

No matter the type of sugar, whether it be white table sugar, honey, syrup, or natural sugar found in fruit, it will all be processed by the body in the same way. Do not be fooled by misleading labelling on food and drink packages, advertising products as containing 'Natural Sugar' or being 'Refined Sugar Free'. This is just a way of encouraging you to buy the product but misleading you to believe that these products are superior from a health point of view. As mentioned before, it is more important to look at the ingredients list and be aware of the sugar added to the products we buy. Ingredients are always listed in order of predominance, with the ingredients used in the greatest amount listed first, followed in descending order by those used in smaller amounts. So if sugar is nearer the top of an ingredients list, it suggests that the product is high in added sugar.

An important thing to note here is that the sugars found naturally in "whole fruit and vegetables and those found in milk and milk products are much better for our health in comparison to natural 'free sugars', such as honey, syrups and unsweetened fruit juices. This is because these foods are considered to be nutrient-dense, providing lots of vitamins, minerals and fibre. They are absorbed more slowly by the body, having a lesser effect on blood sugar levels and they can keep us feeling fuller for longer. Honey, syrups and unsweetened fruit juices are still natural foods. However, they lack many other nutrients and are therefore a concentrated source of sugar, so should only be consumed in moderation.

HOW DOES THE BODY USE CARBOHYDRATES?

No matter which type is consumed, all carbohydrates are broken down and absorbed into the bloodstream in the form of glucose. Glucose is then absorbed by all our cells, with the help of hormones, to be used for energy. Excess glucose which is not used for energy will be stored in the body in the form of glycogen. Glycogen is the stored form of carbohydrates found in our liver and muscles. It is an important reserve source of fuel and can be broken down to form glucose to provide an energy supply during times of low blood sugar levels. The most common situations in which the body uses its glycogen stores for energy is when you have gone a number of hours without eating anything or if you have completed a hard exercise session and have used up all your readily available glucose. This reserve supply of energy is not infinite, so when we go for long periods of time without the ingestion of carbohydrates, we are often left feeling tired, anxious, dizzy and weak. Headaches are also common because the brain does not have any glucose to use as a fuel source. This is why it is important that we consume nutrient-dense, complex carbohydrates regularly in our diet every day, to provide the body with a slow release of energy, keeping our reserve supply of glycogen for when we really need it.

STOP CARB SHAMING

Carbohydrate shaming has been happening for years, which has resulted in many people trying to limit or exclude them from their diet completely, believing wrongly that they are a direct cause of weight gain. This is not the case and is something that everyone needs to understand.

As a result of this misinformation, some claim that low carbohydrate diets are an effective method for achieving weight loss, however these rigid diets are rarely sustainable. Many people don't realise that any weight loss is due to an energy deficit created by eliminating a nourishing food group, which is the main concept that all fad diets share. Plus, some of the weight loss will be due to fluid loss, rather than any significant reduction in body fat. Your body stores some water alongside glycogen, so if you consume a low-carbohydrate diet, you will not only be depleting your glycogen stores, but the stored water that goes along with it.

As mentioned above, we get the energy in our diet from macronutrients. We will discuss energy balance later in more detail in the Calorie chapter of the book; however, it is worth noting here that any extra energy consumed through food and drink will be converted into fat, no matter the source. So, weight gain is not due to the carbohydrate food itself but is related to the amount of carbohydrates consumed.

It can be very easy to eat too much, and it is this overconsumption of any food which can lead to us gaining body fat.

Because of this, it is important to have an awareness of appropriate portion sizes for all foods. Not only that, it is never a good idea to over-restrict any one food group – including carbohydrates. It is this restriction which often makes it more difficult to achieve a balanced diet overall which puts your health at risk.

CARBOHYDRATE MYTH BUSTING

Given that carbohydrates are the body's preferred source of fuel, many people believe that if they restrict their carbohydrate intake, they will trick their body in to using fat as their main fuel source, leading to fat losses and resulting in weight loss. Without sufficient carbohydrate in our diet, our bodies convert fatty acids into energy to meet the demands of our brain, other tissues and organs. This causes ketones to be produced (by-products of fat breakdown), which can have serious side-effects. It is very rare that you would have insufficient carbohydrate in your diet unless you are chronically malnourished with low carbohydrate stores, or if you are following an extremely low carbohydrate diet which is also lacking in protein. Our brains favour using glucose for energy therefore, if we don't include enough in our diets, then our brains have to adapt to using ketones. While this adaptation is happening, the body can also start to breakdown its own protein stores in order to provide an additional source of fuel. Muscles are our richest stores of protein in the body, so if protein breakdown begins, this could lead to the loss of valuable muscle tissue. This is why very low carbohydrate diets are not recommended. By unnaturally switching the body's preferred energy source to fatty acids, people not only tend to report a lack of energy but also that they feel generally unwell. This is likely because with the restriction or elimination of carbohydrates, they are removing what is essentially a very nutrient dense source of food which is important for their overall health and well-being.

So remember, if you are trying to lose weight, the restriction or elimination of carbohydrates will not aid fat loss or weight loss if you continue to eat to your energy requirements by the consumption of other nutrients. It is an overall calorie deficit that must be created rather than the elimination of a particular food group.

HOW MUCH CARBOHYDRATE SHOULD WE EAT?

This is something I get asked so often. Although very low carbohydrate diets are not generally recommended, our portion sizes have increased dramatically in recent decades. Many of us need to be more 'carbohydrate aware', by aiming to have appropriate portions of complex carbohydrates and limiting our overall intake of simple and free carbohydrates. As a general rule, an appropriate mealtime portion of complex carbohydrates, is roughly about the size of your fist. This can be further adjusted depending on your activity levels. According to scientific nutrition experts, around half of our energy intake should come from complex carbohydrates and we should be consuming wholegrain varieties whenever possible.

GLYCAEMIC INDEX OF CARBOHYDRATES

When discussions about carbohydrates arise, the topic of Glycaemic Index (GI) is usually brought up for debate, too. The GI is a rating system for foods containing carbohydrates, showing how quickly each food affects our blood sugar levels when that food is eaten on its own. This is because different carbohydrate-containing foods are digested and absorbed at different rates by the body.

High GI carbohydrates are those which are broken down quickly by the body and cause a rapid increase in blood glucose. Examples include; sugar and sugary foods, sugary soft drinks, white bread, potatoes, white rice, etc.

Low or Medium GI carbohydrates are those which are broken down more slowly by the body and cause a gradual rise in blood sugar levels over time. Examples include; some fruit and vegetables, pulses/legumes and wholegrain foods, such as porridge oats and wholegrain bread.

Although the GI can give us a good idea of the impact a carbohydrate-containing food has on our blood sugar, it should not be used on its own as a method for determining how healthy a carbohydrate-based food is. This is because not all foods with a low GI can be considered 'healthy' and not all foods with a high GI are necessarily 'unhealthy'. For example, watermelon and parsnips are actually classified as high GI foods, while chocolate cake has a lower GI value. Fruit and vegetables are foods that we should consume regularly because they provide lots of nutrients such as vitamins, minerals and fibre. Chocolate cake on the other hand, is something that we should enjoy in moderation because it is high in free sugars and also likely to be high in saturated fat. This difference in the GI rating is because foods that also contain other nutrients such as fat, protein and fibre, actually slow down the absorption of carbohydrates, lowering the GI. Various cooking methods can also impact the GI, as well as the processing and the ripeness of fruit and vegetables. So, focusing on GI alone is not recommended because if you only aim to eat foods with a low GI, your diet may be unbalanced as well as high in fat and energy, which could lead to weight gain. It is for this reason more important for you to focus on the amount of carbohydrates you consume rather than on just the GI, as portion sizes have been found to have a greater influence on blood sugar levels.

Many people also wonder if choosing low GI foods can assist with weight loss. Given that low GI foods result in a slower rise and fall of blood sugar, resulting in a slower release of energy, they can potentially keep you feeling fuller for longer. In addition, low GI foods often contain other nutrients which can also increase a feeling of fullness. Therefore, low GI foods could help control your appetite and may be useful if you're trying to lose weight. However, it is also essential to look at food as a whole and to consider what other nutrients it provides you with, as well as being aware of appropriate portion sizes.

GI AND DIABETES

There are two main types of Diabetes that most of us are familiar with; Type 1 Diabetes and Type 2 Diabetes. However, there are a number of other forms of diabetes, including gestational diabetes, maturity-onset diabetes of the young (MODY) and Wolfram Syndrome.

Individuals with diabetes must be aware of their blood sugar levels. As mentioned previously, when we consume carbohydrate foods, our bodies break them down to form glucose which, in turn, causes a rise in our blood sugar levels. When this happens, an organ in the body known as the pancreas, releases a hormone called insulin. Insulin essentially acts as a transporter, necessary to carry the glucose into all our cells so we can use it for energy. As the cells absorb and use this glucose, blood glucose levels subsequently start to fall. In an individual without diabetes, this decline in blood sugar level is well-controlled by other hormones, making sure that it doesn't go too low and stays within a normal range.

Now, with a focus on the most common types of diabetes (i.e. Type 1 and Type 2), this hormonal mechanism of maintaining blood sugar levels is hindered.

Type 1 Diabetes is an autoimmune condition affecting approximately 10% of people with diabetes in the UK. It is more common in children and teenagers; however, it can occur at any age. This condition causes the body to attack the cells in the pancreas which produce the insulin hormone, meaning the body does not produce any insulin at all. The cause of this remains unknown, so the condition cannot be prevented by lifestyle changes. Individuals with Type 1 Diabetes still break down carbohydrates into glucose, but when the glucose then enters the bloodstream, there is no insulin to transport it into cells. As a result, it cannot be used for energy. Instead, the glucose remains in the blood, causing blood sugar levels to rise over and above the normal range. People with Type 1 Diabetes must therefore inject themselves with insulin on a regular basis in order to manage their blood glucose levels.

Type 2 Diabetes is a condition whereby either 1) the pancreas cannot make enough insulin or 2) the insulin made in the pancreas does not work properly. Either way, the lack of effective insulin causes blood sugar levels to rise. About 90% of people with diabetes in the UK have Type 2 Diabetes. It tends to occur more commonly in adults over the age of 40, however, year after year, more and more young people are being diagnosed. The risk of developing Type 2 Diabetes is related to aging but is also associated with obesity, physical inactivity, a family history of the condition, high blood pressure and if you are of South Asian, African-Caribbean or Black-African descent.

In both conditions, if glucose cannot be taken into the body's cells to be used for energy, many people often experience symptoms of tiredness. With this excess glucose being left in the blood, the kidneys have to do more work to filter it out. This draws a lot of water with it which usually results in an increased need to urinate and increased feelings of thirst, in turn, increasing the risk of thrush (a yeast infection). Other symptoms of diabetes can also include prolonged wound healing (associated with an increased risk of infection) and unintentional weight loss. It is important to be aware of these symptoms so the condition can be diagnosed early and appropriate measures can be put into place to manage it. This is especially important with regards to the possible onset of Type 2 Diabetes, because initially the symptoms may not be severe or obvious since the body is still able to produce some insulin. It is thought that 6/10 people have no symptoms when they are diagnosed with Type 2 Diabetes and may have actually been living with the condition for a while but were unaware of it. Being aware of symptoms is very important because continuous high blood sugar levels over a long period of time can result in serious damage to a number of vital organs and body tissues, including the heart, eyes, feet and kidneys. However, with prompt and correct treatment and care, the effects of diabetes and high blood sugar levels can potentially be reversed or certainly managed.

There are many factors which could contribute to the development of Type 2 Diabetes, but it is not an inevitable part of getting older. As it is not an autoimmune condition and can be related to lifestyle factors, we have an opportunity to help prevent it from developing. It is believed at present that around 3 in 5 cases of Type 2 Diabetes can be prevented or delayed with adopting and maintaining good lifestyle habits.

Given that diabetes requires a focus on controlling blood sugar levels, it is useful to understand the GI, because eating foods with low GI ratings can help control blood sugar levels. However, GI shouldn't be the only thing taken into account. Research has shown that the amount of carbohydrates you eat, rather than their GI rating, has the biggest influence on blood sugar levels after meals. It's also advisable to eat a healthy, balanced diet that is low in fat, sugar and salt, and high in fruit and vegetables.

If you are concerned about your risk or feel you need further advice regarding diet and diabetes, speak to your GP to get a health check and ask about being referred to a Dietitian.

My Tips

To Reduce the Risk of Developing Type 2 Diabetes

» **Eating well**

Eating a well-balanced diet and being aware of portion sizes. Limit consumption of simple & free sugars and limit alcohol consumption. Choose nourishing, wholegrain complex carbohydrates.

» **Moving more**

Try to move every day, whether it be taking the stairs, parking the car further away from your destination, walking more or taking part in some form of exercise.

» **Maintaining a healthy weight**

CHOOSING CARBOHYDRATES

All foods have a place in the diet, and no food should be considered as inherently 'good' or 'bad'. It is clear that there are certain types of carbohydrates which are considered better for our health than others and therefore should be included regularly in our diets, and others which should be consumed less often and enjoyed in moderation.

Our goal should be to consume nutrient-dense, complex carbohydrates in our diet daily to fuel our bodies properly and provide us with additional nutrients such as vitamins, minerals and fibre. Complex carbohydrates should make up the majority of our carbohydrate intake.

Simple carbohydrates are those we should try to consume less often in our diet. They can be divided further into either natural or refined sugars and we also need these in varying amounts, too. Some of the simple carbohydrates which contain natural sugars are food products which include additional nutrients such as protein, healthy fats, vitamins, minerals and fibre which are all beneficial to our health. These should be consumed regularly, but we should remain mindful of our intake because they still contain sugar. The remaining natural simple carbohydrates are those which would be classified as 'free sugars' and we should be limiting our overall consumption of these. Refined simple carbohydrates are unnatural and processed, and also contain 'free sugars'. We should be limiting our intake of these and only enjoying them in moderation.

In order to help simplify this somewhat complex topic, a table has been provided below to give examples of carbohydrate-based foods from each of the categories to make it clearer which foods should be consumed more or less often.

Complex Carbohydrates	Simple Carbohydrates (Natural)		Simple Carbohydrates (Refined)
Aim for complex carbohydrates to make up the majority carbohydrate intake.	Aim to include these carbohydrates regularly in your diet as they provide additional nutrients.	Aim to limit overall consumption of these sugars as they are classified as 'free sugars'.	Aim to limit consumption of these carbohydrates. They are processed and refined, contain 'free sugars' and lack many additional nutrients.
• Wholegrain bread	• Fruits	• Maple syrup	• White table sugar
• Wholegrain rice	• Vegetables	• Agave nectar	• Soft drinks
• Wholegrain pasta	• Milk	• Coconut sugar	• Treacle/Molasses
• Quinoa	• Dairy products	• Honey	• Sweets/Candy
• Oats	• Dried fruit	• Fruit Juice**	• Chocolate (although darker chocolate with a higher cocoa percentage has less sugar)
• Legumes (e.g. lentils, beans and peas)			• Cakes/Pies/Puddings
• Starchy vegetables (e.g. sweet potato, parsnip, potato, butternut squash, corn)			• Refined grains (e.g. white bread, pasta, rice)
			• Biscuits/Cookies
			• Ice cream
			• Sauces
			• Sugary breakfast cereal
			• Fruit juice from concentrate
			• Flavoured yoghurts
			• Golden Syrup
			• Glucose
			• Corn Syrup

FRUIT JUICE**

Although they contain some vitamins and minerals, I generally do not recommend consuming fruit juices, for many reasons. During the juicing process, the natural sugar is released from the cells of the fruit. This means that fruit juices are actually classified as containing 'free sugar', the type of sugar we should be aiming to limit our consumption of. The fibre content is also reduced, meaning fruit juices don't tend to contribute much to satiety levels. This can mean you are more likely to feel hungry soon after drinking it compared to eating a portion of whole fruit. The sugar content per portion of fruit juice also tends to be higher because of this reduction in fibre content and also because you need more than one piece of fruit to make up a serving size of fruit juice. Drinking fruit juice can therefore cause a quick rise and fall of blood sugar levels (and subsequently energy levels), particularly if taken on an empty stomach. Fruit juice also provides additional calories which, if taken in excess, can contribute to an overconsumption of energy. Although fruit juices provide some vitamins and minerals, only one glass of fruit juice (150ml) per day will contribute towards the five portions of fruit and vegetables we are recommended to consume each day. It doesn't matter whether you drink five different types of fruit juice in a day, they will still only contribute to one of your 5 daily portions. This is because fruit juice and smoothies don't contain the fibre which is found in whole fruit and vegetables.

Fruit juice also contains sugar that can damage teeth. It's best to drink them with a meal as this can help protect your teeth against decay. The sugars found naturally in whole fruit are less likely to cause tooth decay because the sugar is contained within the structure of the fruit. When fruit is juiced or blended, the sugars are released, which can cause damage to teeth if consumed regularly.

If I am having a fruit juice, I prefer to make my own in the form of a smoothie. This means I have perfect control over how much fruit I add, and I can also throw in additional healthy ingredients to help reduce the total sugar content. For example, I love to add oats, seeds, vegetables, nut butters, etc. to my smoothies to make a more nourishing and satisfying drink.

FIBRE

Fibre (otherwise known as non-starch polysaccharides, i.e. NSP) are the edible parts of plant-based carbohydrates which are resistant to digestion and absorption in the small intestine. Fibre is unlike the other carbohydrates discussed (i.e. complex or simple) because it is not digested to provide energy but instead it passes into the large intestine (colon) where it is then completely or partially broken down by gut bacteria.

Fibre is considered an essential nutrient for many reasons. It helps with the normal functioning of the gut helping to form stools which are easy to pass through the digestive tract. Fibre is also used as a fuel source for our gut bacteria, which are important micro-organisms needed for digestion and which also play an important role in our immune function. Fibre can help you feel fuller for longer which can also help you maintain a healthy weight, and it has also been associated with a reduction in blood cholesterol and blood pressure levels. Not only that, but a diet that is rich in fibre can also improve insulin sensitivity as this can help slow the absorption of glucose. These health benefits can reduce our risk of a number of chronic diseases, such as cardiovascular disease, type 2 diabetes and bowel cancer.

There are two main types of fibre: soluble and insoluble fibre, which describes the fibres' solubility in water.

SOLUBLE FIBRE

Soluble fibre absorbs water in the gut which can help soften stools, making them easier to pass and reducing the risk of constipation. Soluble fibre includes natural fibres such as pectins, gums and beta-glucans. Sources include foods such as oats, barley, bran, beans and pulses/legumes, fruit, root vegetables and flaxseeds.

INSOLUBLE FIBRE

Insoluble fibre doesn't absorb water and so passes through our gut undigested. It adds bulk to our stools which helps to push other food through our gut. Insoluble fibre includes natural fibres such as lignin and cellulose. Sources include wholegrains, edible skin on fruit and vegetables, as well as nuts and seeds. It is worth mentioning here that if you have diarrhoea, you should avoid insoluble fibre in the short term because it reduces the gut transit time (i.e. the time it takes for food to pass through the gut).

HOW MUCH FIBRE DO WE NEED?

In the UK, the recommendation for fibre for the average adult is 30g per day, however research has shown that the average intake is only about 60% of this i.e. around 18g. For this reason, we should all be aiming to increase our fibre intake whenever possible. Choosing to consume food sources included in the examples already described above can be a good start but it can also be useful to know how to read food labels in order to identify which foods are considered high in fibre.

A food product is: 'high fibre' if it contains at least 6g of fibre per 100g and is considered a 'source of fibre' if it contains at least 3g of fibre per 100g.

Now this does not mean that we all should be counting every gram of fibre we consume. It is simply to encourage people to be more mindful of their food choices and to try and choose higher fibre options whenever possible.

To help put the grams of fibre into context, the table below has been provided to help show how small changes to your diet can help you reach the recommended 30 grams of fibre per day.

Food	Portion Size	Grams of fibre/portion approx.)
Oats	50g	5g
Banana	80g	0.9g
Raspberries	80g	2.5g
Linseeds	7g (approx. 1 tbsp)	1.9g
Apple	1 medium size	2g
Wholegrain bread	2 slices	6g
Baked beans	80g	3g
Almonds	30g	2g
Wholemeal spaghetti (boiled)	100g	3.5g
Broccoli (boiled)	80g	1.8g
Carrots (boiled)	80g	2.0g

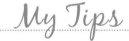

On How to Increase Your Fibre Intake

» Switch to a higher fibre breakfast cereal.

» Add fruit on top of your breakfast cereal or toast.

» Add more vegetables to your diet e.g. through smoothies, soups and homemade sauces (e.g. bolognese, curry, chilli).

» Add fruit, nuts and seeds to yoghurt as a delicious snack.

» Choose wholegrain varieties of food where possible. During the processing of food products to make them white (e.g. white bread and white rice etc.), the fibre content is reduced.

» Choose unprocessed food as much as possible and avoid refined, packaged foods.

» Include fruit and vegetables as a snack, e.g. banana, apple, carrot sticks and hummus.

» Leave the skin on your fruit and vegetables.

» Add more legumes to your meals, e.g. lentils, beans, chickpeas, etc. They can be added to stews, curries, chillies, salads, etc. Check out the recipe section and see how often I include these in the ingredients!

Please remember that with any dietary changes you decide to make, you should always make them gradually and, the same applies to increasing your fibre intake. Increasing your fibre intake too quickly can cause you to experience bloating and gas as your gut tries to adapt to the higher intake. Consider focusing on just one meal or snack at a time; do that for a couple of days and see how you feel. Then move onto adding more fibre to the next meal or snack and continue to build on this gradually. It's also important to remember that if you are increasing your fibre intake, you must also ensure you are staying well-hydrated to allow the fibre to function properly. Keeping active can also help to improve your digestive tract functions.

PROTEIN

Protein is another essential macronutrient that we need to include regularly in our diet. Proteins are known as the building blocks of the human body and can be found in every single cell. They play a vital role in building and repairing body tissues, supporting organ function, and as the enzymes needed for metabolism. Proteins are also essential for efficient hormone and immune function. Our bodies are constantly recycling proteins, so the protein that we eat should considered as so much more than just a nutrient we need in order to fuel our muscles.

Proteins contain essential and non-essential amino acids which are the smaller units that make up proteins. There are 21 different amino acids which can make up different types of protein. It's often useful to describe amino acids as letters of the alphabet. Similar to combining different letters to make different words, we can combine different amino acids to make different proteins. Foods which are considered high in protein contain varying combinations of these amino acids.

Essential amino acids are those that our body cannot make on its own and so they must be obtained from the foods we eat. A complete protein is a protein source which contains all 9 of the essential amino acids. These tend to be animal-based, however there are a few plant-based sources which contain all essential amino acids, too.

Although it's important that we obtain the essential amino acids through our daily dietary intake, we don't have to worry about trying to eat them at every meal. It's just about being mindful of eating a wide variety of proteins to ensure we get an adequate amount of amino acids every day.

Animal Sources of Complete Protein	Plant-based Sources of Complete Protein
• Meat	• Quinoa
• Fish	• Buckwheat
• Eggs	• Soybean
• Poultry	• Hemp seeds
• Milk & dairy products	• Chia seeds

Incomplete proteins on the other hand, are those which don't contain all the essential amino acids. For example, red lentils are a rich source of plant-based protein, but they only contain 8 of the 9 essential amino acids. The majority of plant-based protein sources are incomplete, meaning people who choose to follow a plant-based diet can be at higher risk of being deficient in these essential amino acids. However, this doesn't necessarily make plant-based protein a poor dietary choice. If we choose to consume a more plant-based diet, it is essential that we combine different sources of plant-based protein in order for the foods to complement one another with regards to their amino acid content. This means that the amino acids of one protein source may compensate for the limitations of the other.

This is known as the complementary action of proteins and can improve the biological value of the meal (i.e. provide a better amino acid content). As a result, vegetarians and vegans are encouraged to eat a wide variety of plant-based proteins in combination. If this is done, there is no reason why the quality of protein cannot be as good as that which is obtained in a diet containing animal protein.

Incomplete Sources of Protein

- Legumes (e.g. beans, peas and lentils)
- Vegetables
- Nuts
- Seeds
- Grains

Easy Ways to Combine Incomplete Proteins to Make a Complete Protein-Rich Meal

» Beans on wholegrain toast

» Peanut butter on wholegrain toast

» Combining grains and legumes e.g. my Lentil and Chickpea Curry with brown rice (see the recipe section for this delicious recipe!)

» Porridge oats made with nut butter

» Hummus with vegetable sticks and wholegrain crackers

HOW MUCH PROTEIN SHOULD WE BE EATING?

There is often a stigma attached to protein intake nowadays, with many people believing that protein is only really necessary for athletes and body builders. This has also led to people believing that if they exercise regularly, they must consume an excessive amount of protein to build and maintain muscle mass. On the other hand, some people are under the impression that eating protein will cause them to become 'bulky' from quick muscle gains. This is not the case, and it is so crucial that we all include regular protein sources in our diets daily, to allow our bodies to grow, repair and stay healthy. Not only that, but diets rich in protein have also been found to improve feelings of fullness and, as a result, may help bring about weight loss.

The amount of protein each of us needs varies, depending on a number of factors, such as age, gender, physical activity levels and whether you are pregnant or breast feeding. This naturally makes it impossible to give an exact value suitable for everyone. However, the British Nutrition Foundation recommends that the average adult should aim to consume approximately 0.75g of protein per kg of body weight per day, based on the governments Reference Nutrient Intake (RNI).

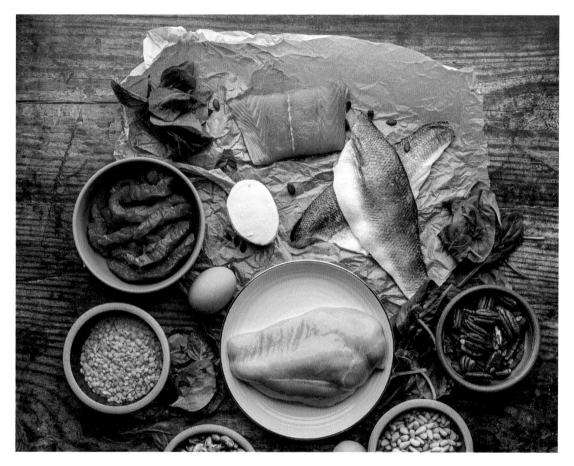

If you are participating in regular sport and exercise, then your protein requirements are likely to be slightly higher than that of the general sedentary population. Extra protein will be required to promote the growth and repair of muscle tissue, improve exercise recovery and prevent muscle protein breakdown. Most people in the UK already consume more than the recommended amount of protein per day, so increasing protein intake by huge amounts often isn't necessary.

We will go into discussing 'Nutrition for Fitness' later in the book, but it is worth noting here that for strength and endurance athletes, protein requirements should be increased to around 1.2-2.0g of protein per kilogram of body weight per day.

It is important to remember that if we don't consume enough protein, the body may break down its existing protein sources to obtain the amino acids it needs to function. Muscle tissue is often a target as it is one of the richest protein sources within the body.

Symptoms of sub-optimal protein intake are not always obvious, but can include

» feeling generally weak and lethargic,

» taking longer to recover after an exercise session,

» dry, brittle and weak hair and nails, and

» reduced immune function (the body is unable to make enough of the proteins used to fight infection/inflammation).

These are some of the more obvious signs of low protein intake. However, given that protein plays a vital role in every cell within the body, there may be other changes in the way our bodies function that we are not aware of.

Contrary to popular belief, higher protein intakes do not equate to more muscle. The body's capacity for storing protein is minimal compared to the way it stores carbohydrate and fat. Once our cells have used all the protein they need from our dietary intake and stored what little they have room for, the remaining amino acids are either converted to glucose or removed from the body in our urine. If we don't need that energy, it will be stored, contributing to excess weight.

Just as it uses the other macronutrients, the body can convert protein to energy if there is a low availability of carbohydrates or fat. However, this tends to be done as a last resort given that protein is needed for so many essential bodily functions.

PROTEIN SUPPLEMENTATION

Following periods of illness, disease, injury or prolonged poor food intake, an increase in protein consumption may be necessary to replenish protein levels and to help restore and improve muscle mass. This can be achieved by increasing the consumption of protein rich foods or by enriching foods with sources of protein (e.g. adding skimmed milk powder to liquid milk rather than water to provide additional protein).

If you have concerns regarding your protein intake or are worried about muscle loss, during or following periods of illness, I recommend you speak to your GP who can assess whether it would be beneficial for you to see a Dietitian and whether the addition of protein supplements is required.

FAT

Fats are the last of the three essential macronutrients that we need in our diet. They provide the body with energy, but they also have so many other important roles and functions within the body. There has been a stigma attached to consuming fat for many years, with many people believing it is automatically associated with weight gain and poor health and we should be completely excluding it from our diet. I do believe that the 'low fat diet' craze is gradually starting to dwindle as more people have become aware of the health benefits of consuming certain types of fat in their diet. However, there are still a lot of misconceptions regarding dietary fat which need to be dispelled.

Many people still hold on to the belief that following a 'low fat diet' is healthier and it will contribute to a greater loss of weight. This is not the case when delicious, real food is being replaced with heavily processed, 'low fat' alternatives that you often see on the supermarket shelves.

Fat is the most concentrated source of energy in the diet when compared to the other macronutrients. This means that if you compare equal portion sizes of a carbohydrate, fat or protein-containing food, the fat source will contain the most calories. One of the reasons that fats have this bad reputation is that they have been automatically associated with weight gain due to being energy dense. Not only that, there are also concerns related to fat consumption being associated with increasing cholesterol levels and having a negative impact on heart health. This section should help clarify this for you and help you to understand the different types of fat, which ones you should aim to choose and how much of them to consume.

WHY WE NEED FAT IN OUR DIET

Fats are found within all the body's cells and have a wide range of important functions within the body.

Fats:

» Provide energy to all the cells in our bodies

» Provide essential fat-soluble vitamins (e.g. vitamins A, D, E and K)

» Provide essential fatty acids (e.g. Omega 3 and 6)

» Provide an insulating layer to help keep us warm

» Provide a protective layer around our vital organs

» Form a structural component of brain tissue and nerves

» Are required for making hormones

» Provide a reserve supply of energy

THE DIFFERENT TYPES OF FAT

There are three main types of dietary fat which we all should be aware of: saturated fats, unsaturated fats and trans fats. Each of these fats have a different structure and it is this which causes them to react differently in the body and have a different impact on our health.

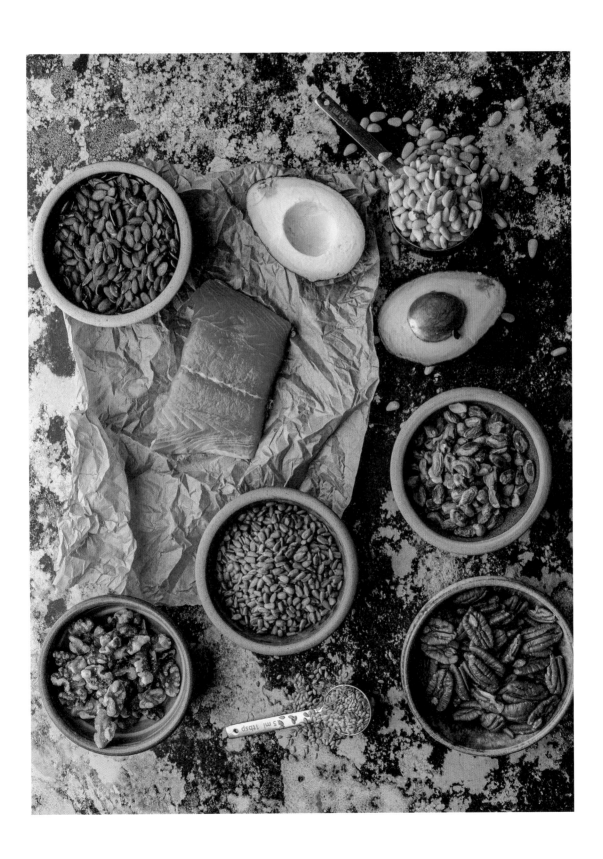

SATURATED FATS

Saturated fats tend to come mainly from animal sources and usually have a solid form at room temperature. Some examples include, butter, meat fat, ghee, lard and dairy products, such as cheese and cream. Other foods that contain saturated fats include, biscuits (otherwise known as cookies in the US), cakes, chocolate and pastries. Foods of plant origin generally have a much lower saturated fat content, although there are some exceptions to this rule. These exceptions include coconut and palm oils, manufactured margarines and fat spreads derived from plant oils.

Saturated fats have been found to increase the total blood cholesterol levels, as well as raise the levels of a certain type of cholesterol in the blood known as Low-Density Lipoproteins (LDL). This type of cholesterol is often referred to as 'bad' cholesterol as it is associated with an increased risk of coronary heart disease. This doesn't mean we need to completely exclude saturated fats from our diet and it is recommended that up to 11% of our total daily energy intake comes from saturated fat. In general, this means that when indulging in foods containing saturated fat, such as when using butter or enjoying chocolate or a piece of steak, we should just be more conscious of the portion sizes we eat and be more mindful of how often we eat them. As the saying goes, everything in moderation. For me, I love butter, chocolate and cakes as much as the next person, and I am a true believer that all food has a place in the diet. Fat adds flavour to food. I often like to refer to foods like these as 'soul food' – food that may not have a lot of nutritional value, but they taste really delicious. I include these types of food in my diet, but I just make sure that I don't eat very much of them, and I don't have them every day.

UNSATURATED FATS

There are two types of unsaturated fats: monounsaturated fats and polyunsaturated fats. They tend to be found in plant-based sources and they both have important functions within the body. Unsaturated fats are believed to be better for our health in comparison to saturated fats. They are not associated with raising total blood cholesterol levels, and some types of unsaturated fats have been found to positively influence the levels of different blood cholesterol types, which can benefit our overall cardiovascular health.

MONOUNSATURATED FATS

These are fats which are typically found in a liquid form at room temperature. The richest sources of monounsaturated fats are olive oil, rapeseed/canola oil, avocados, nuts and seeds. A diet rich in monounsaturated fats has been found to reduce the amount of LDL (or 'bad') cholesterol in our blood, while, at the same time, helping to maintain High-Density Lipoprotein (HDL) cholesterol levels. HDL cholesterol is considered 'good' because it has an important role in transporting 'bad' cholesterol to the liver for removal from the body. This also means that HDL cholesterol may help reduce total cholesterol levels. This can reduce our risk of developing some diseases, such as coronary heart disease and Type 2 Diabetes. For this reason, choosing fat sources rich in monounsaturated fats are thought to be the better fat choice for our health.

POLYUNSATURATED FATS

There are two different types of polyunsaturated fat, known as Omega-3 and Omega-6. These are considered 'essential' meaning that they must be obtained through the diet and are often found in plant-based foods. Omega-3 and Omega-6 fats have different functions in the body, including optimising immune functions, regulating the body's inflammatory processes and promoting normal blood clotting.

Omega-3 fats are found in oily fish, as well as in nut and plant oils, such as rapeseed/canola, walnut, soybean and flaxseed oils. Omega-3 fats have many beneficial functions in the body. They have been found to help maintain normal blood cholesterol levels, have anti-inflammatory properties and anti-thrombotic effects (reducing the formation of blood clots). These beneficial effects can help to reduce the risk of coronary heart disease, as well as other inflammatory diseases such as rheumatoid arthritis and inflammatory bowel disease. Omega-3 fats are also involved in the healthy development of the brain and eyes in unborn children and infants. Further evidence is also emerging suggesting that Omega-3 fats may be effective for maintaining good memory function and also for the prevention and treatment of depression. The richest source of Omega-3 fats are oily fish and the current recommendation is that 2 portions of fish should be consumed per week, 1 portion of which should be oily.

Omega-6 fats are mainly found in vegetable oils such as sunflower, safflower, corn, groundnut, rapeseed/canola and soya oils. They can help to reduce total blood cholesterol levels and, as a result, are thought to be a healthier alternative to saturated fats. However, although Omega-6 fats can help reduce total cholesterol levels and LDL cholesterol levels, excessive consumption can also reduce the levels of good HDL cholesterol. Having low levels of HDL cholesterol is considered to be an independent risk factor for poor cardiovascular health, so we should be mindful of our overall Omega-6 intake. In addition, high amounts of Omega-6 fats are associated with an increased inflammatory response in the body. Although inflammation is essential to survival, i.e., protecting our bodies from infection and injury, an excessive inflammatory response has been linked to cardiovascular disease and cancer. Therefore, we should also be mindful of our intake of Omega-6 fats in the diet, including them only in moderation but making sure that our intake is not excessive. Over recent decades, the Western diet has been shown to generally include more Omega-6 fats due to the increased consumption of vegetable oils and spreads which are rich in these. As a result of the associated increased inflammation associated with high intakes of Omega-6, in the UK it is generally recommended to reduce the intake of Omega-6 fats and instead, choose more Omega-3 options where possible.

So to simplify a somewhat complicated topic, our goal should be to:

»   Limit our intake of saturated fats

»   Choose unsaturated fats where possible, particularly sources of monounsaturated fats

»   Include sources of Omega-3 fats regularly in the diet

»   Include sources of Omega-6 fats in the diet but be mindful of our overall consumption

CHOLESTEROL

Cholesterol is a lipid (fatty substance) which is made in the body by the liver and is considered essential to life. It is a major component of cell membranes and also plays an important role in the production of bile acids, hormones and vitamin D. Cholesterol cannot be dissolved in water and must be transported in the blood attached to proteins. This combination of cholesterol + protein has different presentations in the blood by appearing in different variations in size. This variation in size brings about the names LDL and HDL cholesterol, and it is this difference in size which causes them to have different reactions in the body. Ideally, we should have low levels of LDL cholesterol, and higher levels of HDL cholesterol, due to the effect that each has on cardiovascular health. That being said, we also want to keep our total cholesterol levels within the recommended range because high total cholesterol levels are also known to be an associated risk for cardiovascular health problems.

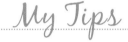

My Tips

To Help Maintain or Reduce Cholesterol Levels

» Keep active

» Follow a healthy, well-balanced diet

» Stop smoking

» Maintain a healthy weight

» Reduce your saturated fat intake and choose unsaturated fat sources instead, particularly monounsaturated and Omega 3 fats (see the following table)

» Eat fewer foods containing trans fats (e.g. biscuits/cookies, cakes etc.)

» Try grilling, roasting, boiling or steaming your food rather than frying

» Trim off all visible fat from meat

» Aim to consume a fibre-rich diet

» Reduce/limit your alcohol consumption

Many people believe that foods containing high levels of cholesterol are those which will have a negative impact on our blood cholesterol levels. It is important to highlight here, that it is actually the type of dietary fat which we consume that actually has a greater impact on our blood cholesterol levels, rather than the dietary cholesterol found in foods. The influence of dietary cholesterol on blood cholesterol levels is generally small unless cholesterol-containing foods are eaten in unusually high amounts. A prime example of this, which I am often asked about, are eggs. Many people are aware that eggs contain cholesterol and so they limit their intake of eggs believing that these will increase their total blood cholesterol levels. This is not generally the case, unless eaten in excessive amounts. Instead, it is rather our saturated fat intake which needs to be limited to help promote better total cholesterol levels. This is because eating high amounts of saturated fat have been found to increase cholesterol levels, particularly that of the 'bad' LDL cholesterol.

Given that there are different types of cholesterol which have very different effects on our health, it can be useful to find out from your doctor what your cholesterol ratio is, especially if you have ever been found to have a high total cholesterol level. Your total cholesterol is made up of both LDL + HDL cholesterol; however, this total value doesn't indicate the amounts of each. Having a higher level of HDL cholesterol is associated with a lower risk of cardiovascular disease. However, it is still important for everyone to avoid having high total cholesterol levels.

If you already know that your cholesterol level is high, or you simply want to avoid developing a high cholesterol level, consider my top 10 dietary and lifestyle tips which can help to maintain healthy cholesterol levels.

TRANS FATS

Trans fats are those we should try to avoid completely. They can be found naturally at low levels in some foods, such as meat and dairy products, but are more commonly found in processed foods such as biscuits, cakes, pastries, margarines and pies. This is because trans fats are created during the manufacturing process of hardening unsaturated fats to form a more solid-spreading fat (e.g. during the manufacturing of margarine). This hardening process is known as 'hydrogenation' and is done to preserve the texture and flavour of the food products, as well as to prolong their shelf life. Although originating as unsaturated fats, trans fats tend to be metabolised by the body in a similar way to that of saturated fats. However, it is thought that trans fats potentially have more detrimental effects than saturates by not only increasing the 'bad' LDL cholesterol but also by reducing the levels of 'good' HDL cholesterol. The use of hydrogenated fats isn't as big a problem anymore in the UK as manufacturers have been trying to reduce the levels of trans fats contained in their products to be more in line with government recommendations for healthy eating. If manufacturers still use trans fats, they must declare this on the food ingredient list so that consumers are informed. The government recommends that adults shouldn't have more than about 5g of trans fats per day. Fortunately, most people in the UK don't eat a lot of trans fats and on average, they eat about half the recommended maximum. In the UK, we tend to eat a lot more saturated fats than trans fats and so we should focus more on reducing our saturated fat intake.

HOW MUCH FAT SHOULD WE BE EATING?

In the UK, it is recommended that total fat intake should contribute to 35% of the total energy intake per day. Of this total, saturated fats should contribute to a maximum of 11% of the total daily

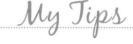

My Tips

For Optimising Your Dietary Fat Intake

1. Choose unsaturated fat options as often as possible

2. Eat more Omega-3 fats

3. Monitor your overall portion sizes of dietary fat (see the section, How to Build a Balanced Plate)

4. Limit your overall intake of saturated fats and enjoy them only in moderation. If choosing saturated fat food, aim to choose good quality options with as little processing as possible.

5. Avoid highly processed food products that contain trans fats.

energy intake. In the UK, the average total fat intake is reportedly close to the recommended amounts, but many people are consuming over the recommendation for saturated fats. We all know that percentages mean very little taken out of context, so instead I like to encourage people to make simple changes to their dietary intake to help meet the guidelines.

QUICK GUIDE TO DIETARY FAT SOURCES

To allow you to quickly check what some of the richest sources are of all the different dietary fats that have been described, this simple table should be helpful.

Saturated Fats	Monounsaturated Fats	Omega-3 Polyunsaturated Fat	Omega-6 Polyunsaturated Fat	Trans Fats
• Meat fat • Full fat dairy • Butter • Coconut and Coconut Oil • Palm Oil • Processed foods	• Avocado • Olive Oil • Olives • Rapeseed/Canola Oil • Nuts • Nut Spreads • Seeds	• Oily fish (e.g. salmon, sardines, mackerel, fresh tuna, herring & trout) • Flaxseed • Walnuts • Chia seeds • Fortified products (e.g. some eggs and yoghurts are fortified with Omega-3)	• Rapeseed/Canola Oil • Corn Oil • Sunflower Oil • Safflower Oil • Peanut Oil • Rapeseed/Canola Oil • Soya Oil • Palm Oil	• Cakes • Biscuits • Margarines • Fried foods • Takeaways • Pastries

A little note about
FISH INTAKE

SUSTAINABILITY

The main source of Omega-3 is from marine fish oil, and it is recommended to consume 2 portions of fish per week, one portion of which should be oily. However, it is known that fish stocks are declining for some species, and for this reason, we should try to choose fish from sustainable sources whenever possible. You can do this by looking for Marine Stewardship Council (MSC) certified products, or looking at The Good Fish Guide from the Marine Conservation Society. In an effort to help with this situation, some of the Omega-3 fats which are being added to supplements are being produced from micro-algae rather than being obtained from oily fish.

Research is continuously being done to try to find sustainable ways to produce plant-based sources of Omega-3.

SAFETY

In recent years, there has been some publicity concerning the chemicals found in some types of fish that may be harmful to humans. Shark, swordfish and marlin may contain concentrated sources of mercury that could be harmful to the developing baby's nervous system and, therefore, consumption of such fish should be avoided by women who are pregnant or planning a baby, and by all children under 16 years of age. For all other adults, including breastfeeding women, the recommendation is that they should eat no more than one portion of these particular fish a week.

Women past childbearing age or not intending to have children, men and boys can eat up to four portions of all other oily fish per week. Women who are pregnant or breastfeeding, or likely to become pregnant, and girls who may become pregnant in the future, can safely have up to two portions of oily fish a week.

WHITE/CANNED FISH

White fish does contain some Omega-3 fats but at much lower levels when compared to oily fish. Nonetheless, white fish does contribute to our intake of Omega-3 fats, which is why the recommendations for fish consumption are that we should aim to consume 2 portions fish per week, one portion of which is oily fish. Some examples of white fish include; cod, haddock, plaice, and red mullet.

Canned fish can also contribute towards our Omega-3 fat intake but usually in far smaller amounts in comparison to fresh fish. It's important to always remember to check the label too, as not all tinned fish will contain Omega-3 fats as they are sometimes removed during the canning process.

SUPPLEMENTS

I am often asked whether someone should consider taking an Omega-3 supplement if they cannot eat fish. Currently, there are no UK recommendations for Omega-3 supplements and it is best to get Omega-3 fats from foods as much as possible, whether from fish or plant-based sources. If you cannot eat fish, focusing on consuming a regular intake of plant-based Omega-3 sources can be useful. Refer to the previous table for examples.

If you choose to take a supplement, it's important to be aware that you need to look for an Omega-3 oil rather than a fish liver oil. This is because fish liver oils contain far less Omega-3 fats and can provide high amounts of certain fat-soluble vitamins, particularly vitamin A. Fish store vitamin A in their livers so by taking a fish liver oil supplement, alongside the vitamin A which can be obtained from your normal dietary intake, you are potentially at risk of consuming too much of this fat-soluble vitamin. The Scientific Advisory Committee on Nutrition advises that if you take supplements containing vitamin A, you should not have more than a total of 1.5mg (1500 µg) a day from food and supplements combined. It's also important to remember that you should not take supplements containing vitamin A if you are pregnant or planning a baby, and always make sure you choose an age-appropriate supplement as children need less vitamin A than adults.

If in doubt, seek advice from a Registered Dietitian.

CALORIES

The amount of energy that an individual needs to obtain from their food intake each day is the amount required to balance their energy expenditure and maintain a body mass ratio which is optimal for good health. Energy expenditure is the energy the body uses to support body functions (e.g. keeping the heart and lungs functioning, etc.) and for body movement. The

A calorie (kcal) is the unit of measurement used to describe the amount of energy we obtain from the food and drinks we consume.

amount of energy required varies greatly from person to person and depends on a number of factors, such as age, gender and physical activity level. This makes it impossible to tell someone exactly the number of calories they need every day.

The body's energy demands are met from the breakdown of the macronutrients found in food. As discussed in the macronutrient section, each macronutrient provides a different number of calories per gram. They also differ in the efficiency with which they provide energy to the body. This means that the body will always breakdown carbohydrates first to provide energy, even in the presence of other macronutrients, because we know that carbohydrates are the body's preferred source of fuel.

Through clinical practice and experience, I know many people who only focus on the number of calories they consume to maintain or lose weight, totally disregarding the types of foods and nutrients that they consume. Just because you are considered to be within a healthy weight category doesn't necessarily mean you are healthy.

I don't believe there is anyone who can honestly say that they enjoy counting calories. Counting calories can take all the enjoyment away from food and can result in an unnecessary restriction on food intake. Many clients I see often admit that counting calories sometimes stops them from taking part in social activities, such as going out for dinner with family or for a coffee and cake catch-up with friends. It shouldn't be that way. No form of eating to maintain health or to help in weight loss should stop you from enjoying time with family and friends.

Given that so many people watch the number of calories they consume, food manufacturers have also started to focus on this from a marketing point of view, labelling foods as 'low calorie' to encourage people to buy them. Having fewer calories does not necessarily make the food healthier. An example that I always like to use for this, is yoghurt. Many yoghurt manufacturers reduce the amount of fat in their products to reduce the overall calorie content (remember, fat contains more calories per gram). However, to make up for the loss of flavour due to the reduction in fat, manufacturers then often increase the sugar content which we also know isn't great for our health.

Although I encourage people to not count calories, I still believe that it is important for everyone to be calorie-aware and to know why the balance of energy is important. The reason for this is that many people think their weight gain is caused by the ingestion of certain nutrients, which is not the case. The cause of weight gain is, in fact, from taking in too many calories, regardless of the macronutrient.

ENERGY BALANCE

The fundamental principle of energy balance, and consequently weight maintenance, can be easily described as follows:

Energy (Calories) In = Energy (Calories) Out

If we consume more calories than what we expend (i.e. calories in > calories out), this will cause weight gain.

If we consume fewer calories than what we expend (i.e. calories in < calories out), this will cause weight loss.

Finding a balance between the two will allow body weight to become stable; however, this doesn't occur on a daily basis, or even a weekly basis, and instead happens over an extended period of time, by eating mindfully and intuitively (see the section on Mindful Eating).

ENERGY EXPENDITURE

Now, I feel it's important to mention here that our total energy expenditure doesn't just come from the energy or calories that we burn through movement or exercise. We actually burn calories in a few different ways, some of which may actually surprise you...

At Rest – We all burn calories, even when at rest, because our heart, lungs, brain and many other bodily functions continue to work, even when we are sleeping or resting. This is known as Basal Metabolic Rate (BMR) – the amount of energy your body needs to function when at rest. If we were to only eat to sustain our BMR, it is quite likely that we would end up feeling unwell, often experiencing symptoms such as weakness and dizziness. We are also more likely to experience more incidences of colds or flu, and some women can also experience loss of their periods. This is because their bodies do not have enough energy to allow menstruation to continue, so the body saves energy by stopping this and gives this energy to essential body functions needed to maintain life (e.g. heart and lung functions). Everyone's BMR is different, depending on body weight, body composition (e.g. levels of fat/muscle tissue), age and gender, pregnancy, disease, etc. It is, therefore, very difficult to calculate this without the use of very expensive equipment. In clinical practice, Dietitians tend to use equations to give a rough estimate of this value.

Eating Food – This is known as the Thermic Effect of Food. Eating requires energy in order to allow the body to digest and absorb the food consumed. This value also varies between individuals and varies depending on the type and portion sizes of food consumed. However, generally speaking, the food you eat only accounts for approximately 10% of total energy expenditure, which isn't very much!

Physical Activity – It is our physical activity levels which make a significant but variable contribution to our daily energy expenditure. This is the thing we have most control over and the one which can have the greatest effect on our energy balance. It varies greatly between individuals, depending on the amount of general bodily movement day to day (i.e. do you spend most of your day sitting at a desk or on your feet?) and also on the type and amount of exercise that you do.

WEIGHT LOSS AND DOING IT RIGHT

For anyone trying to lose weight, a safe way to do this is to eat roughly 500 fewer calories a day or burn 500 extra calories through exercise, or a combination of the two. This is considered a safe calorie deficit, one which will encourage a gradual, more sustainable weight loss of approximately 1-2 lbs per week. Doing anything more excessive than this is likely to be unsustainable in the long run and potentially dangerous for your health.

Eating for your estimated energy requirement every day with no regard to the nutrients you consume does not make you healthy. When discussing energy balance with my clients, many people have the idea that they can eat whatever foods they like, and that as long as they stay within their calorie target, they will still lose weight. This would work if a diet made up of chocolate or cakes was completely satisfying. Think how easy it is to overeat on food products such as chocolate, biscuits and crisps, etc. – we rarely can just eat a few mouthfuls and feel like we have had enough. For this reason, it is pretty unlikely that we would stick to a calorie deficit needed for weight loss on a diet made up of highly processed foods. If we fuel our bodies right with a combination of complex carbohydrates, protein, healthy fats, fruit and vegetables, etc., this will help us feel fuller for longer, thereby reducing the risk of over-eating, while at the same time providing the essential nutrients we need to function at our best.

I believe that, for the most part, it can be beneficial for people to at least have an awareness of calories as well as an understanding of which foods and drinks their main calorie intake comes from. However, I usually suggest that it goes no further than this, but instead actively encourage people to forget the idea that they have to count calories to be healthy and lose weight.

What I encourage you to do instead is to try and pay attention to the nutritional quality of your diet rather than just focusing on the quantity of calories you consume. This means focusing on the number of different nutrients you can provide your body with every day, such as nourishing, complex carbohydrates, high-quality protein, healthy fats, and fruit and vegetables. By eating mindfully, having an awareness of appropriate portion sizes and nourishing your body with delicious, wholesome foods, you are far more likely to feel satisfied by your food intake and unlikely to over-eat.

Understanding why it's important for your health to include certain foods in your diet is far more rewarding than only focusing on the number of calories you consume. Focus more on the inclusion, rather than the exclusion, of certain food, choosing food that you know will give you energy and nourish your body at the same time.

I always say that the best diet is one you know you can stick to for the long-term. For anyone who asks my advice on a new diet that they are considering starting, I always ask the following three questions:

1. Do you think you will be able to stick to it long-term?

2. Do you think you will actually feel happy following it?

3. Will it provide the right amount of nutrients, as discussed throughout this book, to nourish your body?

If the answer to any of these questions is no, I must encourage you to think about why you are thinking of following that diet in the first place.

The way I encourage my clients to nourish their bodies is to create a balanced plate, including food sources from all the main food groups, based on recommended portion sizes, rather than counting the number of calories. The section on Building a Balanced Plate will follow our discussion on the importance of Micronutrients.

MICRONUTRIENTS

Micronutrients are nutrients which the body needs only in small amounts, ('micro' meaning small). They include nutrients known as vitamins and minerals, which are considered to be 'essential', meaning the body is unable to make its own supply of these and so they must be obtained through our dietary intake. There are a number of different kinds of vitamins and minerals in our diet, all required in varying amounts and all playing very different vital roles and functions in the body. Consuming a diet with a wide range of animal and plant-based foods is key to making sure we get enough of each. If we are able to do this, then it is often not necessary to take supplements.

VITAMINS

There are 13 vitamins that we need to include in our diet, 4 of them are considered fat-soluble and 9 are considered water-soluble. Fat-soluble vitamins (able to be dissolved in fat) are vitamins A, D, E and K. Water-soluble vitamins (able to be dissolved in water) include the B-vitamins and vitamin C. Water soluble vitamins cannot be stored in the body and excessive intakes tend to be excreted by the body in our urine on a daily basis. Fat-soluble vitamins can accumulate in the body if taken in excess and, as a result, can potentially have a negative impact on our health. For this reason, before thinking about taking a vitamin supplement, you should consult your doctor or a registered Dietitian for advice.

Fat-Soluble Vitamins

Vitamin	Function	Source
Vitamin A	Considered an anti-oxidant. Required for the normal renewal and repair of body tissue (e.g. skin) and plays an important role in reproduction, embryonic development and growth. Essential for ensuring good vision in dim light and important for maintaining a good immune system.	• Liver and liver products • Fortified margarine and fat spreads • Dairy products • Oily fish • Egg yolk • Fish liver oils • Dark green leafy vegetables • Orange-coloured fruit & vegetables
Vitamin D	Works in helping the body to absorb Calcium which helps keep bones strong. It also plays a role in optimal muscle function and maintaining a good immune system.	• Skin exposure to sunlight • Oily fish • Meat, particularly liver • Eggs • Dairy products • Fortified foods
Vitamin E	Considered an anti-oxidant. Prevents damage to body cells.	• Vegetable oils • Nuts & seeds • Fat spreads and margarines
Vitamin K	Required for the normal clotting of blood. Also plays an important role in kidney function and in the formation of bone.	• Dark green leafy vegetables • Vegetable oils (e.g. rapeseed, soybean and olive oil) • Smaller amounts in meat and dairy products.

Water-Soluble Vitamins

Vitamin	Function	Source
Vitamin B1 (Thiamine)	Required for the release of energy from food. Plays an important role for the normal functioning of the nervous system.	• Fortified breakfast cereals • Meat and meat products (especially pork) • Vegetables • Pulses • Nuts • Wholegrain bread • Eggs
Vitamin B2 (Riboflavin)	Required for the release of energy from food and for normal growth. It helps maintain healthy skin and eyes and is needed to support the function of the nervous system.	• Milk and dairy products • Eggs • Green leafy vegetables • Meat and meat products • Fortified breakfast cereal
Vitamin B3 (Niacin)	Required for the release of energy from food. Plays an important role in the functioning of the nervous system and in keeping skin healthy.	• Meat and meat products • Fortified wholegrain and cereal products • Fish • Nuts and seeds • Eggs • Milk and dairy products • Yeast extracts
Vitamin B6 (Pyridoxine)	Required for the release of energy from protein and carbohydrates. Helps to form red blood cells which carry oxygen throughout the body.	• Fortified breakfast cereals • Meat and meat products • Bananas • Nuts • Pulses/Legumes • Wholegrain products • Fish • Bread • Eggs • Vegetables • Milk

Vitamin B7 (Biotin)	Required in small amounts to help breakdown fat.	• Egg yolk • Liver and kidney • Nuts • Pulses/Legumes • Wholegrain cereals
Vitamin B9 (Folate/Folic Acid)	Helps the body form healthy red blood cells. Reduces the risk of central neural tube defects, such as spina bifida, in unborn babies.	• Leafy green vegetables • Milk and dairy products • Pulses/Legumes • Oranges • Fortified breakfast cereal
Vitamin B12 (Cobalamin)	Required for making red blood cells and keeping the nervous system healthy. Needed for releasing energy from food and allowing the body to use folic acid.	• Meat and meat products • Fish • Milk and dairy products • Eggs • Fortified breakfast cereal
Pantothenic Acid	Required for releasing energy from food.	Found widely in a large variety of plant and animal foods, especially: • Green leafy vegetables • Meat • Eggs • Peanuts
Vitamin C	Considered an anti-oxidant. Assists in the absorption of iron and helps to protect cells from damage. Helps to maintain healthy skin, bones, teeth and gums and helps maintain immune system and nervous system functions.	• Berries and currants • Citrus fruits • Strawberries • Broccoli • Potatoes

MINERALS

Like vitamins, we also need minerals in small amounts as they play an essential role in the normal functioning of the body. There are approximately 8 main minerals we need in our diet, in addition to 6 main trace elements (other minerals that are needed in much smaller amounts). There are additional trace elements which are known to be present in the human body, but there is limited evidence that there is a dietary requirement for them.

The following table describes the 8 main minerals and two important trace elements that we need to be aware of.

Minerals

Mineral	Function	Source
Calcium	The most abundant mineral in the body. Considerable amounts are required to create and maintain our bone structure. Also important for maintaining healthy teeth and for the normal functioning of nerves and muscles. It also helps blood to clot normally.	• Milk and dairy products • Fortified cereal and cereal products • Green leafy vegetables • Tahini and sesame seeds • Pulses/Legumes • Fish containing soft bones • Breads using fortified flour
Phosphorus	Essential for building and maintaining strong bones and teeth and for helping to release energy from food.	• Milk and dairy products • Meat • Fish • Eggs • Nuts • Bread and wholegrains
Magnesium	The second most abundant mineral in the body. Plays a vital role in skeletal development, normal muscle and nerve function. Helps to release energy from food.	• Wholegrain Bread • Meat and meat products • Nuts and seeds • Dairy products • Green leafy vegetables • Fish • Wholegrain cereals

Sodium	Plays a vital role in fluid balance within the body.	• Small amounts are found naturally in foods. Sodium tends to be high in sources where salt is added during processing. • Processed meats • Smoked fish • Cheese • Butter • Salted food (e.g. nuts and biscuits) • Savoury snacks • Ready meals
Potassium	Plays an important role in fluid balance and the normal functioning of muscles and nerves. Helps maintain normal blood pressure.	• Potatoes • Fruit (especially bananas, citrus fruits, apricots) • Mushrooms • Pulses/Legumes • Chocolate • Coffee • Malted milk drinks • Tinned and packaged soups • Nuts and seeds • Meat • Fish • Wholegrain breakfast cereal
Iron	Plays an important role for carrying oxygen throughout the body. Required for obtaining energy from food. Helps maintain a healthy immune system and brain function.	• Red meat • Liver and offal meats • Fortified bread and cereal products • Green leafy vegetables • Pulses/Legumes • Nuts and seeds • Dried fruit • Wholegrain products (e.g. brown rice)

Zinc	Required to build muscle and for hormone production. Needed for processing carbohydrates, protein and fat in food. Helps maintain normal hair, skin and nails and assists with the healing of wounds. Supports normal fertility and reproduction.	• Red meat • Fish and shellfish • Milk and milk products • Poultry • Eggs • Bread • Cereal products
Fluoride	Needed for maintaining strong bones and teeth and helps prevent tooth decay.	• Tap water • Tea • Toothpaste
Iodine (Trace Element)	Essential mineral for thyroid function and for the production of thyroid hormones. Needed for the maintenance of our metabolic rate, body temperature regulation, protein production and maintaining connective tissue. It's also important for brain and central nervous system development.	• Fish and shellfish • Sea salt • Dried seaweed • Eggs • Milk and dairy products
Selenium (Trace Element)	Helps maintain the normal functioning of the immune system. Prevents damage to the cells in our body and is also needed for the production of thyroid hormones.	• Bread • Meat products • Poultry • Fish • Nuts • Eggs

Although there are many vitamins and minerals that we need to include in our diet, they are generally needed in such small amounts that we often consume enough without having to try too hard. Vitamins and minerals are available from a wide variety of both animal and plant-based food sources, which means that if you consume a varied and well-balanced diet, you should be able to get all the micronutrients you need. My personal recommendation is that people should aim to consume a wide variety of colour in their diet when it comes to choosing fruit and vegetables. Different colours tend to suggest a different nutrient source so, as the saying goes, 'eating the rainbow' is a really great way to help optimise our nutrient intake. The only exception to this is if you have been diagnosed with a specific deficiency and have to ensure adequate amounts of that nutrient.

SALT INTAKE & HEALTH

Sodium is a component of common salt, otherwise known as Sodium Chloride. Sodium is responsible for regulating body fluids and electrolyte balance. Too much salt in our diets can cause health problems such as water retention (a build-up of fluid in the body which can cause tissue to become swollen) and high blood pressure. High blood pressure increases the risk of heart disease, kidney problems and strokes. Blood pressure is simply the pressure that is exerted on the walls of the blood vessels and arteries. Arteries are the large blood vessels that carry the blood from your heart to your brain and to the rest of your body. A certain amount of pressure is needed to keep the blood circulating through your body. High blood pressure, otherwise known as hypertension, means that your blood pressure is consistently higher than the recommended level. It often has no symptoms, and it is thought that as many as 7 million people in the UK are living with undiagnosed high blood pressure without knowing they are at risk. Over time, high blood pressure can cause damage to your blood vessels and put you at a greater risk of cardiovascular disease.

It is believed that many people in the UK have high blood pressure as a result of consuming too much salt in their diet. This is thought to either be because they are adding too much salt to their food, or because they are consuming a lot of food products which have had lots of salt added during processing.

Nutrition experts recommend no more than 6g of salt per day for healthy adults; however surveys have demonstrated that many people in the UK still exceed this recommendation by up to a third more. For this reason, it can be really beneficial to read food labels to help you choose foods which are lower in salt (see section, Food Labels).

As well as looking at food labels, there are also many other ways you can help lower your salt intake.

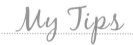

To Lower Your Salt Intake

» Add salt either during cooking or at the table, not both and if using, only use small amounts.

» Try using other herbs and spices to season your food instead.

» Cut down on salty processed foods and ready-to-eat meals and try and make your own food if you can. This way you are in control of the salt added.

» Ask in restaurants and takeaways for no added salt.

» Be wary of gourmet salts and salt substitutes claiming to be better for your health than table salt – these products are still likely to add some form of salt to your diet and are often higher in other ingredients which are best to avoid.

SALT 'VS' SODIUM

To confuse us, some food labels may only state the sodium content of the product. It's important that we don't mix up the two.

To convert sodium to salt, you need to multiply the sodium content by 2.5.

For example, 1g of sodium per 100g is 2.5 grams of salt per 100g.

Adults should have no more than 2.4g of sodium per day, which is equal to 6g of salt.

It's also worth noting here that there isn't always an explanation for the cause of high blood pressure, as often many lifestyle factors can play a part. Other lifestyle factors which can increase the risk of high blood pressure include: lack of physical activity and exercise, being overweight or obese, drinking too much alcohol or having a family history of high blood pressure.

CALCIUM & VITAMIN D FOR BONE HEALTH

Most of us know that we need calcium to maintain strong bones and teeth, but I believe bone health is an area of nutrition which is often overlooked and not given the attention it deserves.

All our bones make up our skeleton which is the main structure that holds our bodies together. We need to take care of our bones throughout our entire lives, to help us continue to function as best we can as we age and to help prevent the onset of bone-related diseases.

Osteoporosis is a medical condition when the body's bones weaken and lose strength, increasing the risk of breaking or fracturing a bone. It tends to develop gradually over a number of years and is often only diagnosed after a bone fracture has been caused from just a minor fall or sudden impact. It is believed that over 3 million people in the UK are affected by this condition, with more than half a million people needing hospital treatment every year for fractures which are likely to be a result of osteoporosis. This medical condition is on the rise, but unfortunately, many people are unaware that they are even affected as osteoporosis tends to show no symptoms until a break or fracture actually occurs.

Losing bone strength is a normal part of ageing, but the speed in which this occurs can be affected by many lifestyle factors. This means we have the opportunity to do something about it.

Women are known to be at a higher risk of developing osteoporosis than men as women tend to lose bone more rapidly following the onset of menopause. However, other risk factors for the condition which affect both men & women include;

» A diet low in calcium and vitamin D

» Lack of regular weight-bearing exercise

» A family history of the condition

» Having a low Body Mass Index (BMI)

» Smoking

» An excessive alcohol consumption

» Certain medical conditions, e.g. inflammatory conditions, conditions associated with malabsorption

» Certain steroids and other medications

It's essential to stress the importance of good bone health from an early age because there is so much we can do to help reduce the risk of this condition from occurring.

Childhood and young adulthood are our bone-building years. As we grow, our bone mass increases until we reach our Peak Bone Mass (PBM), which is defined as the highest level of bone mass achieved as a result of normal growth. The age at which PBM is achieved varies but is normally reached in the late teens or early twenties. Once PBM has been achieved, bone mass is thought to remain relatively stable until the age of approximately 45-50 years. Then, after a decline in male and female hormones, bone loss begins to occur gradually. Therefore, if we 'build up' plenty of bone mass during childhood and early adulthood, our bones will be in a better position to withstand the loss of bone mass as we get older.

PBM can be affected by genetics, gender and race, however, there is still a large component of PBM variation that is determined by modifiable environmental factors. Although all the risk factors noted above are considered to be important, research has found strong evidence supporting a positive effect of calcium intake and physical activity on bone accumulation and growth. As a Dietitian, my concerns lie in the fact that many children and young adults aren't consuming a nutritionally adequate diet or aren't doing enough physical activity to support their bone health. Eating disorders are also on the rise, which can have a serious impact on an individual's bone health, as a result of a poor nutritional intake, or low body weight.

From a description of all the vitamins and minerals noted above, it is clear that it is not just calcium that has an impact on our bone health. Many other nutrients also play a vital role, including vitamin D, vitamin K, vitamin C, Phosphorus, Magnesium and Fluoride. Therefore, achieving good bone health concerns so much more than just consuming lots of dairy products. Even though Calcium is the most abundant mineral in our bones, to ensure good bone health, we need to make certain that we also get these other nutrients in our diet, too. For example, even if you consume a calcium-rich diet, without enough vitamin D you cannot absorb the calcium properly. Whilst some of our vitamin D can be obtained from dietary sources, there are not many vitamin D-rich foods and our richest source actually comes from the exposure of our skin to sunlight. Unfortunately, it can be challenging for us to get enough vitamin D from the sun, particularly for those of us living in the UK. As we all know, the weather and the hours of daylight we get in the UK are pretty unsatisfactory at times, particularly during the winter months. For this reason, nutrition experts recently changed the vitamin D recommendations for those living in the UK in order to help ensure we are getting enough. The advice is now as follows:

• **Between late March/early April and September**, the majority of people aged 5 years and above will probably obtain sufficient vitamin D from sunlight when they are outdoors, in addition to consuming foods that naturally contain or are fortified with vitamin D. As such, they **might choose not to take** a vitamin D supplement during these months.

• **From October to March** everyone over the age of five will need to rely on dietary sources of vitamin D. Since vitamin D is found only in a small number of foods, it might be difficult to get enough from foods that naturally contain vitamin D or fortified foods alone. So everyone, **should consider taking** a daily supplement containing 10 micrograms (10µg) of vitamin D.

(British Nutrition Foundation, 2016)

So, despite there only being a small number of vitamin D-rich foods, dietary sources are still considered essential, especially when exposure to sunlight is limited. It is also worth noting here that taking a vitamin D supplement, as well as eating foods rich in vitamin D and spending a lot of time outside in sunshine, is not a problem. However, we must be careful not to take more than one supplement which contains vitamin D as the 10-microgram recommendation could be exceeded. Remember, vitamin D is a fat-soluble vitamin, meaning it can be stored in the body if it is consumed in excess. The supplement should also be appropriate for the age group or medical condition and should also be the right dosage. Many supermarkets and health food shops sell vitamin D supplements which contain more than the 10 microgram recommendation. If you are unsure, I would always recommend speaking to your doctor or a Registered Dietitian before buying any supplements.

Nonetheless, it is absolutely crucial that we get enough calcium in our diet to optimise our bone health. The guidelines for the amount of calcium we need per day can be found in the following table.

Calcium Recommendations	
Age Group	Calcium (mg) per day
Young Children (1-10 years)	350-550mg
Teenage Girls (11-18 years)	800mg
Teenage Boys (11-18 years)	1000mg
Adults (19 years+)	700mg
Breast feeding Women	1250mg
Women after menopause	1200mg
Osteoporosis (Adults)	1000mg

Out of context, I'm aware these amounts can mean very little, so I have provided a list of calcium-rich foods to help you reach your daily target.

Food	Quantity/Portion	Calcium Content (mg)
Dairy Sources		
Milk	200ml	240mg
Cheese	30g	220mg
Yoghurt	120g	200mg
Rice Pudding	200g	176mg
Custard	120ml	120mg

Calcium Fortified Non-Dairy Sources		
Calcium-enriched milk alternatives (e.g. soy, oat, nut)	200ml	240mg
Calcium fortified cereals	30g	130-150mg
Soy-bean curd/tofu (Only if set with calcium chloride or calcium sulphate not nigari [magnesium chloride])	60g	200mg
Calcium-fortified bread	1 slice (40g)	191mg
Calcium-fortified soya yoghurt/ dessert/custard	125g	150mg
Non-Dairy Sources		
Sardines (with bones)	60g	258mg
Tinned salmon (with bones)	52g	47mg
Wholemeal bread	2 x slices (100g)	54mg
Broccoli (boiled)	2 x spears (85g)	60mg
Spinach (boiled)	120g	180mg

These are just a few examples of different foods that contain calcium, but there are many other sources available. Hopefully this helps to illustrate that your calcium target can actually be met through food alone, and it doesn't necessarily need to come just from dairy products. Think about including calcium sources at your meals, or even as a snack to make sure you are getting enough.

Despite many bone health benefits resulting from nutritional intervention measures being made from a young age, it's also important to remember that it's never too late to start making changes. Even after a diagnosis of osteoporosis, the benefits of nutritional intervention can still help to prevent further loss of bone mass.

HYDRATION

Water isn't actually classified as a nutrient as such, but we do need to consume plenty of it every day to stay healthy. Water makes up about 60% of our body, yet many of us do not drink enough in order to stay well-hydrated.

Water has many functions in the body. One of its most obvious roles is to regulate body temperature. It is also required for transporting nutrients and other compounds through the blood, removing waste products through urination, and acting as a lubricant and shock absorber for our joints. Every day we lose water through urination and sweat, as well as small amounts through respiration and through our skin. If we are not replacing all the water we lose with fluids from the food and drinks we consume, we can easily become dehydrated.

Given that about two-thirds of our body is made up of water, drinking water is the best way to stay well-hydrated. However, other fluids that provide water can also contribute towards hydration levels, too, such as tea, coffee, milk, fruit juices and soft drinks. If we decide to consume these types of fluids, we should be mindful of their energy, sugar and caffeine contents and aim to consume them only in moderation, with water making up the majority of our total fluid intake. If you struggle to drink enough water, choosing decaffeinated fluids, and low or reduced sugar options will also contribute to your fluid intake without adding a significant number of additional calories.

Food can also contribute to our fluid intake, usually contributing about 20% of our total water intake. Fruit and vegetables are largely made up of water and so are foods such as soups and stews, etc., which usually have a lot of water added during the cooking process. Alcoholic drinks do not contribute towards hydration, as alcohol is considered a diuretic – something that causes you to urinate more.

Staying well-hydrated is important for so many health reasons. It helps with the removal of toxins and waste products from the body and can help prevent urinary tract infections, constipation, skin problems, kidney stones, headaches and dizziness, to name but a few. It is also important for preventing fatigue and maintaining good concentration levels and it also plays a major role in exercise and performance by improving endurance levels. Keeping ourselves well-hydrated can also help regulate appetite, making it far less likely for us to reach for something to eat when our body doesn't necessarily need it. It's very common for the brain to confuse thirst with hunger, unless you are experiencing physical thirst, and in that case you would already be dehydrated. This can result in our eating, rather than just replacing the fluid we need. Thirst is only part of the way hydration is regulated in the body, and it's important to remember that when you drink, it's common to stop feeling thirsty before your body is completely rehydrated. I always encourage getting plenty of fluids regularly throughout the day, both at meal times and in between, to stay well-hydrated and to help manage our appetites.

HOW MUCH WATER DO WE REALLY NEED?

The frustrating answer – it's impossible to give an exact amount that is suitable for everyone. This is very dependent on age, weather, physical activity and sweat loss, etc. The general recommendation is to consume about 6-8 glasses a day. This equates to a daily goal of approximately 1600mls for the average adult female and about 2000mls for the average adult male. However, this may need to be increased if the weather is hot, if you are exercising, or during periods of acute illness (e.g. if you are experiencing diarrhoea).

The best way to tell if you are well-hydrated is to actually monitor the colour of your urine. When the body detects that it is dehydrated and that it needs more water, the first thing that happens is that the kidneys reduce the amount of water that leaves the body in the urine. This means that the colour of the urine becomes darker. If you are drinking enough, your urine should be a pale yellow colour.

I always encourage people to think about getting a reusable water bottle to help keep track of their intake. I love a water bottle that is designed to keep my water cool throughout the day, as I personally find water more challenging to drink if it's lukewarm. Drinking water, which is refreshingly cold, often with the addition of some fruit to flavour it, can really help to increase your daily intake. Another tasty alternative is to drink decaffeinated fruit teas which can be lovely served cold, too.

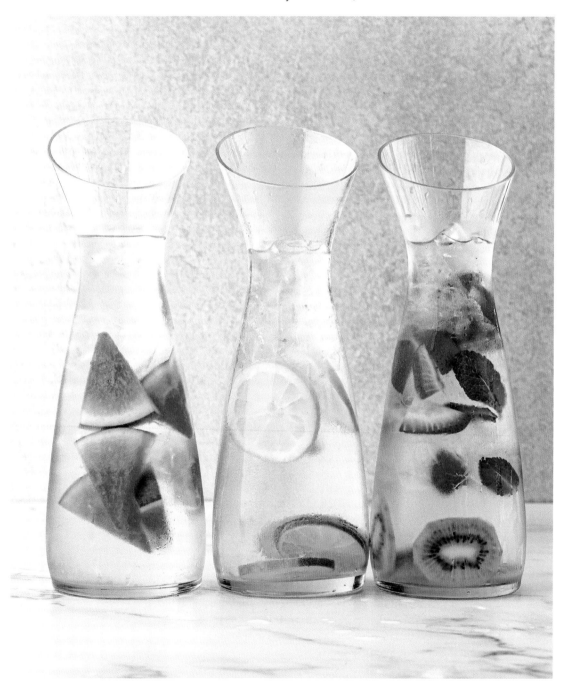

I always like speaking from personal experience when it comes to hydration too. Despite always being on my feet while working and exercising regularly, too, I used to be someone who was guilty of not drinking enough. So, I decided to set myself a challenge several years back to try to drink at least 2000ml every day. I knew that to make this a habit, I'd have to commit for at least three weeks. It was difficult, but I love a challenge and honestly, I cannot tell you how much better I felt afterwards. I was much less fatigued, I felt stronger in the gym, I had more endurance and was more comfortable on my runs, and I was able to concentrate more during lectures, studying, and at work. Not only that, my skin became so much clearer, it looked less tired and dry, and I experienced fewer breakouts. I will admit, for the first few weeks, I did have to run to the toilet more often than usual, but this gradually reduced as my body became more efficient at dealing with this higher volume of water. Now that my body has adapted and expects this level of hydration, I feel really encouraged to continue drinking to this volume, as it can make me feel so sluggish when I don't.

CAN WE DRINK TOO MUCH?

It is possible, although drinking too much is very rare. It usually occurs only in individuals with certain medical conditions, for example, those which effect heart, liver or kidney functions. If you do drink fluid in excess amounts and your body cannot get rid of the excess quickly enough, the sodium levels in your blood can become dangerously low. This can have serious health consequences. It is unlikely to happen under normal conditions but has actually happened in individuals who were following a very extreme detox programme.

Building a Balanced Plate

I get it. You are probably thinking how on earth is it possible to make sure you are eating enough to fuel your day, while at the same time making sure you are including every nutrient we have just learned about without it becoming a full-time job? Don't worry – I've got your back. With the information I have given you so far, you now have the knowledge and the power to be able to make healthy choices when it comes to food shopping and preparing meals. It can be a lot of information to take in, but remember, you don't have to get it right all at once, and certainly no one gets it right 100% of the time – even me.

Life is far too short to count calories. Remember, reaching your calorie requirement every day doesn't necessarily make you healthy. Instead, I would encourage you to focus on eating food from a variety of different food groups every day which, in turn, will help you to include all the essential nutrients.

There are five main food groups that we should consider:

1. Protein

2. Complex Carbohydrates

3. Healthy Fats

4. Fruits and Vegetables

5. Dairy or Dairy Alternatives

By building your plates based on these food groups and trying to eat a variety of different food sources from each group, you should be able to get all the nutrients you need in order to stay healthy and fuel your day. When it comes to portion sizes, rather than weighing your food, I encourage people to use their hands to get a rough idea of an appropriate serving size. This is never going to be 100% accurate but it can be a simple, easy and useful way of helping to ensure you are getting the right portion sizes. Let's talk about how you do this.

STEP 1 – PROTEIN

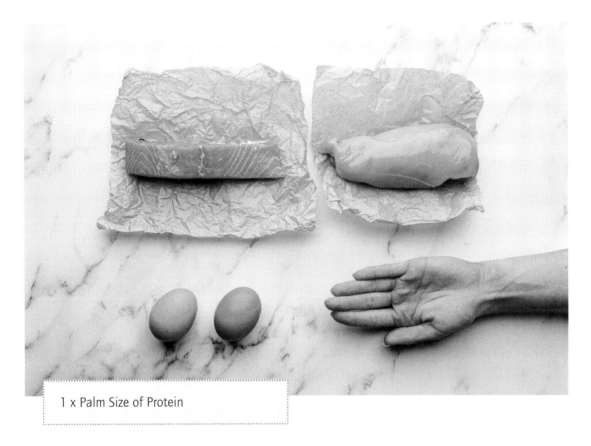

1 x Palm Size of Protein

In the protein section, I mentioned that everyone has different protein requirements that depend on different factors, such as age, gender and physical activity levels. I personally eat towards the higher end of the protein requirement recommendations. I am very physically active, so I need the extra protein for building and repairing muscle tissue. Not only that, but I also find protein foods really filling which helps keep me feeling fuller longer. Because of this, I usually tend to base my meals around protein-rich foods. I know that if I include a protein source in each of my main meals, as well as in my snacks, then I will roughly be hitting my higher protein target without having to measure anything in grams. For an individual who has a higher body weight, and therefore a higher protein requirement, it is likely that 2 palm-sized servings of protein consumed regularly throughout the day would better meet their protein goals. To help put this into perspective, here is a little example of how I try and hit my protein target every day:

Meal	Portion Size	Protein Serving
Breakfast	50g oats	5g
• Porridge oats made with milk	150ml milk with oats	5g
• Coffee with milk	250ml milk with coffee	8g
Snack	1 tbsp peanut butter	3g
• Peanut butter (eaten with 1 apple, sliced)		
Lunch	200ml lentil soup	5g
• Lentil soup & rye crackers	4 x rye crackers	4g
Snack	30g nuts	7g
• Nuts		
Dinner	1 medium chicken breast	30g
• Chicken breast		
Supper	100g Greek yoghurt	10g
• Greek yoghurt with handful of nuts	30g nuts	7g
	TOTAL PROTEIN	84g

In this example, I have only listed the main protein sources eaten at each meal and snack. The total amount of protein does not include that which would also be obtained from other incomplete protein sources that would be included at each meal and snack, too, such as some fruit and vegetables and a source of complex carbohydrates, etc. Remember, this is only a rough estimation, but hopefully it helps to illustrate that hitting high protein targets can be achieved through the consumption of food alone, without the need for any protein supplements (protein supplements are covered later in the 'Nutrition for Fitness' section).

STEP 2 – COMPLEX CARBOHYDRATES

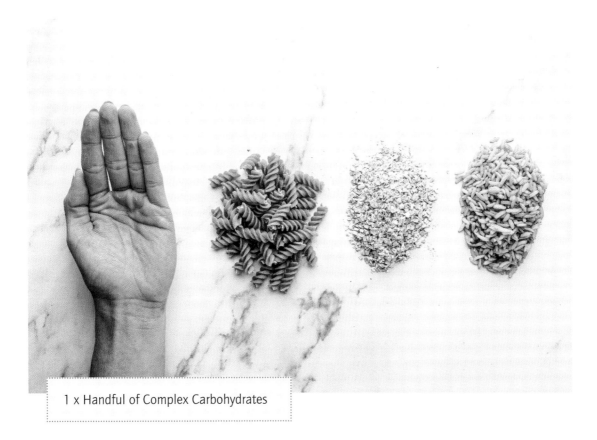

1 x Handful of Complex Carbohydrates

After reading about carbohydrates in the nutrition section, I hope this has helped you to understand why you need to include complex carbohydrates regularly in your diet and that they should not be a forbidden food group. I mentioned earlier what people tend to do wrong is that they consume too large a portion of carbohydrates. By using your hands again as a measuring aid, you can make sure your portion size is appropriate. One handful size of complex carbohydrates gives you a rough idea of an appropriate portion size to include at each meal. If you are a physically active person, you might need a second handful to meet your energy needs. Remember too, that complex carbohydrates don't just provide you with slow-releasing energy, they are also great sources of fibre and lots of vitamins and minerals. Include at least one serving at each meal, depending on your energy needs, and always choose the unprocessed, wholegrain varieties whenever possible.

STEP 3 – FRUITS & VEGETABLES

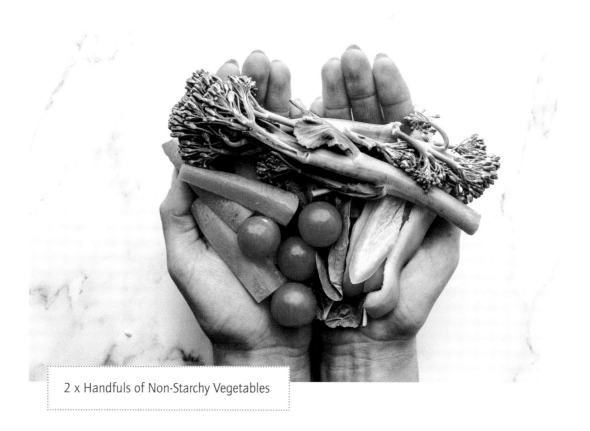

2 x Handfuls of Non-Starchy Vegetables

Non-starchy vegetables include foods such as spinach, peppers, carrots, mushrooms, broccoli, green beans and leafy green vegetables. Vegetables are generally low in calories and provide lots of vitamins, minerals and fibre. We should try to include at least 2 handfuls of non-starchy vegetables at mealtimes, choosing a variety of different-coloured options to optimise our nutrient intake. I personally do my best to include 2-3 different vegetable sources in my meals, particularly for lunch and dinner, and I always try to fill up at least a third to a half of my plate with these.

Starchy vegetables, such as parsnip, potatoes, butternut squash, pumpkin and sweet potatoes, are not included in this group due their higher carbohydrate content and should be portioned as a complex carbohydrate.

I think it is important to mention fruit here, too, given that I mentioned fruits and vegetables are actually considered one food group. Fruit was discussed in the Carbohydrate section and is described as a source of natural, simple carbohydrates. I mentioned that simple carbohydrates can be included in our diet, but we need to be aware that they contain sugar and as a result, we should be mindful of our portion sizes and how often we eat them. However, I also said in this section that sources of whole fruit, although being a source of simple carbohydrates, also include many other nutrients, such as fibre, vitamins and minerals.

This means that they are not only a very nourishing food choice, but with these additional nutrients, whole fruit also tends to have a lesser impact on blood sugar, and they can also help keep us feel fuller for longer. For this reason, whole fruits should be included regularly in the diet but are not something that we generally recommend to be taken in larger portions at every meal, like with non-starchy vegetables. I would, therefore, recommend a portion size of fruit as being either one piece of whole fruit, such as one banana, one orange or one apple etc., or equivalent to 1 handful (i.e. approximately 80g). Personally, I tend to prefer a sweeter breakfast, and for those of you who follow me on social media, you know how much I love my porridge and fruit in the mornings. Otherwise, the rest of my daily meals are made up of lots of non-starchy vegetables, and I tend to include a piece of fruit as a healthy snack between my meals, if I feel I need it. Therefore, I always aim to reach the recommended 5 portions of fruit and vegetables a day by having the majority of these come from non-starchy vegetable sources.

STEP 4 – HEALTHY FATS

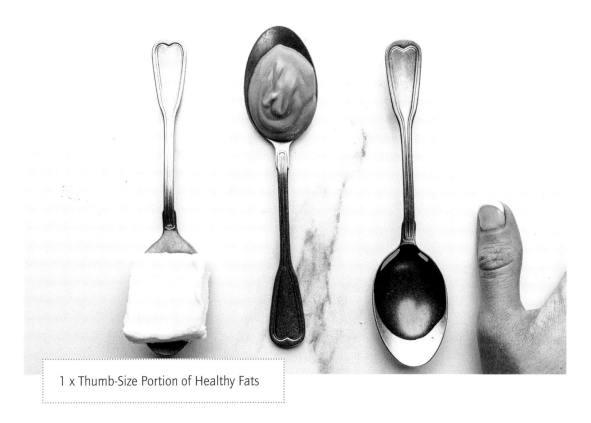

1 x Thumb-Size Portion of Healthy Fats

I mentioned in the Fat section that there are some fats which are considered better for our health than others. I also highlighted that although it is good to include these fats in our diets to help prevent cardiovascular disease, all fat, no matter what kind, is energy/calorie dense. For this reason, it is important that we aim to choose the healthier kinds of fat whenever possible, but still remain mindful of the portion size we consume. A rough idea of an appropriate serving size of fat is the size of your thumb. I like to include healthy fats as a little addition to my meal, for example, by using some oil to cook with or to drizzle over salads, using half an avocado to spread on toast or to chop up and put in salads, or having some nut butter to stir into my porridge or dip my apple slices into as a snack. Remember, healthy fats not only bring nutritional benefits, but they also add flavour to food, too. Simply by being mindful of your portion sizes, you can boost the nourishment that a meal or snack provides without adding an excessive number of calories to your energy intake.

STEP 5 – DAIRY & DAIRY ALTERNATIVES

Dairy and alternatives are considered the last of the food groups. Dairy foods provide the richest and best absorbed source of dietary calcium, however, there are other non-dairy sources of calcium which can contribute greatly to our overall calcium intake.

Dairy, or a suitable alternative, doesn't necessarily need to be included at every meal, but it is important that we include calcium rich food sources throughout the day, either through meals or snacks. I encourage clients to aim for at least three portions per day which should meet most calcium requirements. The amount of calcium varies hugely depending on the portion size of dairy product or alternative. This makes it harder to determine an appropriate serving size for this food group. Instead, I would recommend looking at the food label itself which usually indicates an appropriate serving size, or have a look at the Bone Health section for examples of different food products that provide a generous amount of calcium to help meet your calcium requirements.

A quick note on soul foods…

Foods that are known to be high in sugar and fat, such as crisps/chips, sweets, chocolate, biscuits/cookies, cakes, etc. are not considered foods which should be included in our diet every day, therefore they are not listed in any of the previously mentioned food groups. This is because food products like these are not considered essential for our bodies to function at their best, mainly because they are known to be nutrient-poor foods, i.e. they provide very little nutritional nourishment to the body but can provide a high number of calories per serving. For this reason, it is advisable to indulge in such foods only in moderation. These sorts of food are foods which I like to call 'soul food'. They might not be the most nourishing for our body in terms of nutrients, but we all know that they can provide delicious enjoyment and sometimes that's what's important.

Dairy products are a source of saturated fat and can therefore be energy dense. Choosing reduced fat versions can help to limit your overall saturated fat intake and can be useful if you are watching your waistline, particularly if you regularly include dairy products in your diet. Reduced fat varieties tend to have less vitamin A and vitamin E than whole milk but have more minerals, such as calcium, potassium and phosphorus. The reason why the vitamin content is lower in the reduced fat versions is because these vitamins are fat-soluble vitamins and as a result, are removed with the removal of some of the fat content. If you are consuming a varied, well-balanced diet, this slightly lower vitamin content is likely to be insignificant.

Food Shopping

HOW TO READ FOOD LABELS

Being able to read food labels can be a great way to help you compare different products and help you to choose the healthier option.

Nutrition information is found on the food label, usually in a table. It usually appears alongside the following information:

» The name of the food

» The weight of the food

» The ingredients in the food product (listed in descending order of quantity used)

» Allergy advice

The following table is an example of a nutrition label on a loaf of bread (revised to remove the list of ingredients, etc.). This is typical of what you will find in the UK.

Ingredients	Nutrition				
Listed in descending order...	Typical Values	100g contains	Each Slice (typically 44g) contains	% RI	RI* for an average adult
ALLERGY ADVICE For allergens, including cereals containing gluten, see ingredients in **bold print**	Energy	985kJ	435kJ		8400kJ
		235kcal	105kcal	5%	2000kcal
	Fat	1.5g	0.7g	1%	70g
	of which saturates	0.3g	0.1g	1%	20g
	Carbohydrate	45.5g	20.0g		260g
	of which sugars	3.8g	1.7g	2%	90g
	Fibre	2.8g	1.2g		
	Protein	7.7g	3.4g		50g
	Salt	1.0g	0.4g	7%	6g

This loaf contains 16 servings.

*Reference Nutrient Intake for an average Adult (8400kJ/ 2000kcal)

All nutrition information is given per 100g of the product but will also sometimes be provided per portion, too. Manufacturers must always provide the nutrition information at least in per 100g to allow easier calculation if the typical serving size is not consumed. Voluntary information can also be given on other nutrients such as unsaturated fats, fibre, and vitamins and minerals. If a product claims to contain a certain nutrient, the amount of the nutrient contained in the product must also be given on the nutrition label. For example, if the product states that it is a 'source of calcium', the amount of calcium it provides must also be noted on the nutrition label.

The information provided in the nutrition label for US products is very similar, as can be seen in the following example. For more specific information on how to read US nutrition labels, visit www.fda.gov.

Nutrition Facts	Amount Per Serving	% Daily Value*	Amount Per Serving	% Daily Value*
Serving Size 2 slices (57g)	Total Fat 2g	3%	**Total Carbohydrate** 29g	10%
Servings Per Container 8	Saturated Fat 0g	0%	Dietary Fiber 4g	16%
	Trans Fat 0g		Sugars 5g	
Calories 140 Calories from Fat 20	Polyunsaturated Fat 1g		**Protein** 7g	4%
	Monounsaturated Fat 0g			
	Cholesterol 0mg	0%		
	Sodium 200mg	8%		
	Vitamin A 0%	Vitamin C 0%	Calcium 6%	Iron 8%
	Thiamin 8%	Riboflavin 2%	Niacin 4%	Folic Acid 6%

*Percent Daily Values are based on a 2,000 calorie diet. Your daily values may be higher or lower depending on your calorie needs.

	Calories	2,000	2,500
Total Fat	Less than	65g	80g
Sat Fat	Less than	20g	25g
Cholesterol	Less than	2,400mg	2,400mg
Potassium		3,500mg	3,500mg
Total Carbohydrate		300g	375g
Dietary Fiber		25g	30g

PACKAGE FRONT LABELLING

Many food manufacturers also include an additional label on the front of the product packaging, which displays key nutritional information using a traffic-light colour-coding system. This is not mandatory for manufacturers, but can be a quick and easy way to display information about the nutrients which are important for our health, e.g. fat, saturated fat (saturates), sugar and salt. This information will either be written per 100g/100ml, per portion or both.

In the UK, these product labels use a traffic-light colour-coding, using the colours red, yellow and green, to quickly show whether a product is high (red), medium (yellow) or low (green) in the particular nutrients displayed. This will help you quickly and easily compare food products and can help you to make healthier choices. When buying a packaged food product, you should try to choose lots of greens, some yellows and only a very few reds.

It is also important to be aware that the portion size determined by the manufacturer may not be the portion size that you actually end up eating. Quite often we actually consume more than the portion size as determined by the manufacturer. To help become more portion-wise, the next time you buy a packaged product, look at the serving size recommended and compare it to the portion size you normally eat.

US food manufacturers are now more frequently including similar food labels on their packages. Though they may not follow the same colour-coding system, the information provided will be similar and should be just as useful.

GUIDELINES FOR FOODS BEING CLASSIFIED AS HIGH, MEDIUM AND LOW

The UK government has provided guidance on levels of total fat, saturated fat, sugar and salt to help determine whether a product can be considered high, medium or low in these nutrients. Being aware of these values can be useful if manufacturers decide not to display the traffic-light colour-code labelling on the front of their product.

My Tip

Take a little photo of this table with your phone so you have it nice and handy whenever you shop for food!

Nutrient	LOW	MEDIUM	HIGH
Total Fat	≤ 3.0g per 100g	> 3.0g to ≤ 17.5g per 100g	> 17.5g per 100g
Saturated Fat	≤ 1.5g per 100g	> 1.5g to ≤ 5.0g per 100g	> 5.0g per 100g
Sugar	≤ 5.0g per 100g	> 5.0g to ≤ 22.5g per 100g	> 22.5g per 100g
Salt	≤ 0.3g per 100g	> 0.3g to ≤ 1.5g per 100g	> 1.5g per 100g

The US government has created a program called MyPlate, which can be found at choosemyplate.gov. They also provide information on the levels of total fat, saturated fat, sugar and salt to help you determine how much should be included in any diet. Visit the site for more information specific to US food products and for understanding US government nutrition guidelines.

HEALTHY, TIME- AND COST-EFFICIENT FOOD SHOPPING

As well as being aware of the nutrition labels when you are choosing a product, there are many other ways you can shop healthier.

Did you know that the more natural, healthier food products (e.g. fruit and vegetables, fresh meat and fish, and fresh bread) are usually found around the outside perimeter of the supermarket? This means that the more processed, refined products are usually found in the middle aisles and shelves of the supermarket. Not only that, but many supermarkets will display special offers on these food products at the end of the aisles or at the checkout to catch your eye. This is good to know if you are someone who is easily tempted when walking past these items. Now you know how to potentially avoid them.

I know that it's not always possible, but I strongly encourage you to not shop on an empty stomach. Shopping when we are hungry usually means we opt for foods which will quickly bring our energy levels back up again, such as chocolate and sweets. When we are hungry, our rational thought processes often go right out the window and we may buy and then eat these foods quickly, consuming a bigger serving size than we might have done otherwise.

Today, most of us lead pretty busy and sometimes hectic lives. A common pitfall is a lack of planning. If we don't plan our food intake for the day or days ahead, we tend to reach for the more processed foods or opt for takeaways. This can be both expensive and unhealthy if it's something we do regularly. Don't worry. It happens to the best of us! The trick is to get organised and spend just a little bit of time each week planning a rough idea of what you would like to eat each day to keep this from becoming a common occurrence. Your food plan doesn't necessarily need to cover everything, but it should cover just enough so that you don't go through every day without any clue about what your next meal will include. Thinking ahead and having a general idea of what you would like to eat over the next few days will also help you plan your shopping list. Then you can have all the ingredients you need to hand to allow you to cook on the day you plan to eat that meal, or food-prep a little in advance to save you time cooking on your busier days.

This leads me very nicely to talking about shopping lists! Anyone who knows me knows I love lists! Making a shopping list is one of the best tips I can possibly give you. I have a regular shopping list in my kitchen noting all the usual food staples I like to keep in my cupboards. Every week, I spend a few minutes checking through my kitchen cupboards to make sure I have everything I need for that week while writing down anything else I need. Doing this helps stop you from buying food items that you don't really need. It's also a good idea to write your list in a way so that all the similar food products are grouped together, (e.g. list all the fruit and vegetables next to each other). This will stop you running from one end of the store to the other to find what you're looking for, as well as reducing the risk of you adding extra food items to your basket that you don't necessarily need.

The following table is an example of the regular shopping list in my kitchen that I refer to every week. It includes those food products that I have to keep at hand most days (e.g. oats, milk, fruit and vegetables, etc.), and it also includes other ingredients that I use regularly and which I like to keep a supply of in my kitchen or in my freezer.

Shopping List

Wholegrain Carbohydrates

- Oats
- Brown rice
- Wholegrain bread or rye bread
- Wholegrain pasta
- Quinoa
- Bulgur wheat
- Wholegrain rice cakes
- Wheat biscuits
- Oatcakes
- Wholegrain crackers

Meat & Fish

- Free range eggs
- Free range chicken breasts
- Salmon fillets
- Lean minced beef
- White fish (e.g. seabass, etc.)
- Tinned tuna (in spring water)

Fruit

- Bananas
- Apples
- Raspberries
- Strawberries
- Blueberries
- Lemons
- Limes
- Dates
- Avocados

Dairy & Alternatives

- Dairy Milk
- Greek yoghurt (or natural with no added sugar)
- Unsweetened almond or oat milk
- Cheese

Fats (Spreads & Oils)

- Grass-fed butter
- Extra virgin olive oil

Vegetables

- Mushrooms
- Tomatoes
- Green beans
- Sugar snap peas
- Rocket
- Spinach
- Peppers
- Frozen mixed vegetables
- Brown onions
- Red onions
- Sweet potatos
- Broccoli
- Carrots
- Potatoes
- Butternut squash
- Spring onions

Seasoning + Herbs & Spices

- All Spice
- Dried Basil
- Bay Leaves
- Ground Cinnamon
- Crushed Chillies
- Chilli Powder
- Dried Coriander
- Curry Powder
- Ground Cumin
- Cayenne Pepper
- Fresh Garlic
- Garam Masala
- Ground or fresh Ginger
- Italian Seasoning
- Mixed Herbs
- Nutmeg
- Oregano
- Paprika
- Dried Parsley
- Rosemary
- Tarragon
- Thyme
- Turmeric
- Sea Salt
- Black Pepper

Legumes

- Red lentils
- Chickpeas
- Kidney beans
- Butter beans
- Black Beans
- Black-eyed beans
- Haricot Beans

Nuts & Seeds

- Nut butter
- Almonds
- Cashews
- Linseeds
- Toasted flaked almonds
- Pumpkin seeds
- Chia seeds

Miscellaneous

- Low-salt stock cubes
- Passata
- Reduced-fat pesto
- Tomato puree
- Tea
- Coffee
- Honey
- Maple syrup
- Baking powder
- Bicarbonate of soda
- Plain flour
- Self-Raising flour
- Wholemeal flour
- Cocoa powder
- Cocoa Nibs
- Vanilla essence
- Desiccated coconut
- Stevia sweetener
- Balsamic vinegar
- Distilled vinegar
- Soy sauce

Organic Food: Should You Be Choosing It at the Shops?

When a food is described as 'organic', it simply refers to how the food was produced. Organic farming is a system which avoids the use of man-made fertilisers and pesticides, growth regulators and livestock feed additives. Organic legislation also generally prohibits irradiation and the use of genetically modified organisms (GMOs).

Organic farming is a system which works towards environmentally, socially and economically sustainable food production, and as a result, food products which are classified as organic, are often higher in price. However, whether this type of farming is more sustainable than conventional farming techniques, remains controversial.

Many people think that organic food is better for our health; however, the evidence for this is limited. It is recommended to thoroughly wash fruit and vegetables with tap water as a great way of removing any pesticide residues.

It is likely that a mixture of organic and other innovative farming systems will be necessary in future to feed the global population without compromising the health of the ecosystems that agriculture relies on. However, from a health perspective, there is no strong evidence to prove that eating organic foods is better for us, so whether you choose to buy organic food is entirely up to you. Personally, I always like to choose organic, free-range eggs and meat from local butchers, as well as buying fish which has been sourced sustainably.

Busting Nutrition Myths

There are so many nutrition myths that make eating healthy very confusing for many of us. The list of diet fads is also so long that the topic alone would need a book of its own. Here I'd like to shed light on a few of the myths we hear about most often.

DETOX DIETS

'Detox' is a buzzword we see everywhere nowadays, particularly on social media. It is short for the word 'detoxification', which is the name given to a process that occurs in the body, whereby organs, such as the liver and kidneys, work to get rid of waste products. Unfortunately, the word detox is often incorrectly used in the health and beauty worlds to describe 'detoxing' your body with the help of supplements or by eating or drinking certain foods. It is particularly common to hear of people doing this after periods of over-indulgence (e.g. Christmas).

There have been many detox products for sale over the years with some more recognisable ones being 'detox' teas, 'skinny' coffee, juice cleanses and colon cleanses. Most of them claim to aid in weight loss, improve hair, nail and skin condition, increase energy levels or improve digestion and the immune system. Sounds good, right? As the saying goes, if it sounds too good to be true, it probably is, and concerning detox diets, that's definitely the case.

The whole idea of detox is absolute nonsense. And I'm being polite here. As I mentioned before, the body is pretty incredible, and it has all it needs already to remove any waste products and toxins (big shout-out to our liver, kidneys, intestines and skin!). Our body constantly filters out toxins and waste products like alcohol, medications, products of digestion and bacteria. There are no pills or specific drinks, lotions or potions that can do that magic job. It is one of my biggest frustrations that often the sales of these products are promoted by celebrities and influencers, who are paid to share them with their large followings on social media. Often those people who look for these quick fixes have no understanding of just how dangerous these products can be for our health. These products can contain ingredients such as laxatives and diuretics. These ingredients may be natural or chemical, but they have the same effect, causing you to go to the toilet more often than you actually need to. You may lose weight following detox diets, but any difference you see on the scales is most likely because of fluid loss. Over time, this can cause you to become dehydrated and depleted in essential nutrients. In addition, detox diets can play havoc with your digestive system and even cause permanent damage to your body. I can only hope that someday the sales and promotion of these unsafe products will be banned.

GLUTEN IS BAD FOR EVERYONE

'Gluten free' is another diet fad that has reared its ugly head over recent years, with beliefs that gluten is bad for our health and should be eliminated from our diets. Gluten is a protein found in cereals, wheat, rye and barley. There is also a similar protein which can be found in oats. Gluten is a natural protein which helps give the lovely texture to dough used to make bread and other similar food products, which many of us know and love.

Most often, the rumours surrounding gluten tend to suggest that it is fattening and harmful to our digestive system. This is not supported by scientific evidence.

Most people can digest gluten just fine but for those diagnosed with coeliac disease or who have a gluten sensitivity, this is not the case and gluten is in fact harmful for them.

Coeliac disease is a serious auto-immune, inflammatory condition which affects the small intestine and occurs as a result of the body having a reaction to gluten. Auto-immune simply refers to a reaction by the body, whereby the body's tissues are attacked by the body's own immune system. In coeliac disease, the body's immune system mistakes gluten as being something harmful and the subsequent reaction results in damage to the surface of our small intestine. Damage to this area of our body in turn impacts the absorption of nutrients from the food we eat. It is therefore important to note that coeliac disease is not an allergy, nor a food intolerance. It is thought that 1 in 100 people in the UK are affected by the condition, which is usually characterized by symptoms such as diarrhoea, constipation, vomiting, stomach cramps, mouth ulcers, fatigue and anaemia. It is diagnosed by blood tests and a tissue biopsy of the small intestine. Both are required to determine a definite diagnosis because blood tests are not always accurate and can sometimes provide negative results despite coeliac disease being present. The only treatment for coeliac disease is a life-long adherence to a strict gluten-free diet. This allows the lining of the small intestine to heal and repair itself after which symptoms should be resolved.

If you think that you may have coeliac disease, I encourage you to go and see your GP for appropriate testing. Don't ignore the symptoms. If left undiagnosed, untreated coeliac disease holds a greater risk of other health complications including anaemia, osteoporosis, neurological conditions, and although rare, there is also an increased risk of small intestine cancer and intestinal lymphoma. This also applies to individuals who have had a confirmed diagnosis of this disease. The strict removal of gluten is essential to help prevent other complications, and this is especially important even if you only experience mild symptoms associated with the condition.

It's worth noting here, too, that some people can also experience unpleasant intestinal symptoms when eating foods with ingredients containing gluten, even if they don't have coeliac disease itself. This is often referred to as Non-Coeliac Gluten Sensitivity (NCGS). The symptoms of this may be similar to those experienced by many people with coeliac disease, but it is not clear if and how the immune system is involved, and there does not appear to be any damage to the lining of the intestine. NCGS is a new area and more research is needed to understand the condition and who exactly is at risk. There are also no specific diagnostic tests for NCGS yet, but it tends to be considered as a diagnosis of dietary exclusion, i.e. coeliac disease has been ruled out, but people experienced an improvement in symptoms after excluding gluten from their diets.

This is where I feel it's important to stress that if you are concerned that you may have coeliac disease or a sensitivity to gluten, you shouldn't cut out gluten before being tested. Anti-bodies (the products of our immune system which help fight against anything considered harmful) are what is looked for in the blood test. If you remove gluten from your diet, your anti-body levels fall dramatically, which means blood tests won't show there is an issue and neither will the results of the small intestine biopsy. It's also so important for me to stress here, too, that you should not exclude gluten from your diet without nutritional guidance from a Dietitian. Cutting out gluten unnecessarily (i.e. with no diagnosis of coeliac disease or gluten sensitivity), without appropriate guidance from a nutrition expert, can put you at a higher risk of nutritional deficiencies, and may also cause you to develop an unnecessary negative relationship with certain foods.

The increased interest – or should I say health stigma? – in gluten over recent years has resulted in more gluten-free products being available on our supermarket shelves. On the one hand, this is great for those who actually need to avoid gluten for medical reasons, but on the other hand, it has caused more people to become aware of gluten and has increased the misconception that gluten is something that needs to be avoided by everyone. As a Dietitian, this is something that I find particularly frustrating as I feel this diet fad has overshadowed coeliac disease, which like I mentioned before, is a serious health condition.

To sum up, if you don't have coeliac disease or you don't have a sensitivity to gluten, you should be perfectly able to digest this natural protein and you do not need to remove it from your diet. Just because you see 'gluten-free' on a food label, doesn't make it healthier. The removal of gluten doesn't mean that the food product is in any way lower in refined sugar, salt, saturated fats or trans fats.

THE KETOGENIC DIET HELPS US BURN FAT BETTER AND LOSE WEIGHT

This diet has had celebrities around the globe trying it and (unfortunately) raising its profile, particularly over the last year or so. The Ketogenic (or Keto) Diet is a diet which is typically very low in carbohydrates (carbohydrates make up around 5% of our total calorie intake per day), relatively high in fat and contains a moderate amount of protein. It tends to involve the exclusion of grains, dairy, legumes, soy products, most fruits, as well as starchy vegetables (e.g. parsnips, butternut squash, etc.). The carbohydrates in the diet, therefore, mainly come from non-starchy vegetables and nuts and seeds.

The idea behind this diet is that by decreasing the amount of carbohydrates you consume, the body switches from burning carbohydrates as its primary energy source, to burning fat. We touched on this in the Carbohydrate section, noting that this dietary change causes increased ketone levels in the body (this is where the diet gets its name), and by doing this, people claim that it can help you to control your hunger, help you to lose weight and help you improve your health. Even more worryingly, some people claim that it can treat or prevent a number of different types of cancer. Again, put politely, this is complete and utter nonsense. Those who make such claims are also likely to believe in another diet myth which claims that sugar 'feeds' cancer cells – therefore effectively speaking, a low carbohydrate diet would 'starve' cancer cells preventing their growth. Unfortunately, it's not that simple. Cancer cells usually grow quickly, which does require a lot of energy, meaning they need lots of sugar. However, cancer cells also need lots of other nutrients, too, such as amino acids and fats, so it is not just sugar they crave. As mentioned previously, all our healthy cells need sugar, too, and there is no way to tell our bodies to let healthy cells have the sugar they need, but not give it to cancer cells. Following restricted diets with very low amounts of carbohydrate could damage health in the long term through the elimination of foods that are good sources of fibre and important vitamins we need for general health and immunity. This is even more important for individuals with cancer. Some cancer treatments can cause undesirable weight loss and put the body under a lot of stress, so having a poor nutritional intake as a result of following a restrictive diet could also negatively impact recovery, or even be life threatening. To achieve weight loss, you need to create a suitable calorie deficit, and this is why the Keto Diet shows results. It is not because you have 'switched' to burning fat as a fuel, but instead it is the result of your creating a calorie deficit by removing a food group (i.e. carbohydrates) that people often tend to eat too much of anyway. Most of the initial weight loss seen is actually more often associated with fluid loss rather than body fat loss.

When starting this diet, people often tend to report symptoms such as low energy levels, increased hunger, sleep problems, nausea, digestive discomfort, bad breath and poor exercise performance. This can make following this diet both unenjoyable and hard to sustain. Restricting or excluding any food group can make it more difficult to achieve a balanced diet. In this case, with the restriction of carbohydrates and dairy products, people lose out on amazing sources of energy, fibre, vitamins and minerals. The Keto Diet is also very high in fat. We discussed previously that it's important to consider exactly what types of fats are being included in the diet, bearing in mind that some fats are better for our health than others.

**NOTE: The only area in which there is evidence that a Ketogenic Diet may provide benefits is with the medical condition epilepsy. It is considered a medical treatment for this condition that should only be done under the supervision of a Dietitian, requiring regular blood monitoring and support due to the side effects associated with it. **

WE MUST EAT FOODS WHICH ARE 'ALKALINE' TO KEEP THE pH OF OUR BLOOD WITHIN THE RIGHT LEVELS

Supporters of this next diet myth claim that by changing the kinds of foods we eat and by consuming more alkaline and less acidic foods, we can help change the pH balance of our blood and as a result, reduce health risks, such as cancer and osteoporosis.

The term 'pH' is a figure that expresses the acidity or alkalinity of a solution and is measured on a logarithmic scale. In this case, we are referring to the pH value of our blood. A pH of 7 is considered neutral, with lower values being more acidic and higher values being more alkaline.

This is another diet that lacks any form of scientific evidence, and sadly is based on a misunderstanding of basic human physiology. The pH of our blood is well-maintained within a very narrow range (between 7.35 and 7.45), thanks to our kidneys, regardless of the type of diet we consume. Any extra acid or alkali is removed from the body by urinating, so all that changes is the pH of our urine, not of our blood. If our bodies failed to keep our blood pH within normal levels, we would know about it very soon and become very ill, very quickly.

The only reason why people see weight loss results from following this sort of diet is simply because it encourages the removal of processed foods from the diet and encourages consumption of fruit and vegetables, but so do all other healthy eating patterns. It has got nothing to do with foods being more acidic or more alkalic.

WE SHOULDN'T EAT AFTER A CERTAIN TIME OF NIGHT

Verdict: Absolute nonsense.

The theory behind this dietary fad is that if we eat food too late at night, it causes us to gain weight because our metabolism slows down as we sleep and so we aren't burning off the energy counsumed.

Your metabolism does slow slightly as you sleep, essentially because there's no need for it to be working as fast as it does during the day when you're moving more and needing the extra energy to get through the day. Although it slows down when you sleep, it's only a slight amount, and your metabolism never actually stops. Think about it – without ongoing metabolism of food or energy stores within the body, how can our heart and lungs, etc. keep going while we sleep?

The only reason why people tend to see weight loss results from following this type of dietary pattern is because they put themselves in a calorie deficit by not eating the foods they would usually eat in the evening, e.g. a supper or extra snacks. It has got nothing to do with our metabolism working any slower.

WE SHOULD AVOID DAIRY PRODUCTS BECAUSE HUMANS DON'T NATURALLY DIGEST MILK FROM ANIMALS AND MILK IS FULL OF HORMONES

The background behind this dietary myth comes from people believing that humans shouldn't be consuming the milk of another animal species and if we do, the milk is pumped full of hormones during the production process and that the consumption of these is bad for our health.

Often the reason why people believe that we shouldn't be consuming cow's milk (or another mammal's milk) is that they believe that we don't naturally have the ability to digest it. This isn't true. The background to this needs a little more explanation, so bear with me.

Milk of any kind, from any mammal, including humans, contains a carbohydrate called Lactose (often referred to as milk sugar). Lactose is a simple sugar consisting of two sugar molecules (glucose and galactose) joined together. Mammals naturally produce milk to support their young, therefore most of us are naturally equipped with the 'lactase' enzyme which is needed to break this sugar down so that we can use it for energy. This means that no matter what mammal the milk comes from, humans have the ability to digest it, as long as they have the lactase enzyme.

In most mammals, the activity of the lactase enzyme decreases after weaning, because milk no longer tends to be the major source of energy in the diet anymore. However, in some human ethnic groups, lactase activity can persist even into adult life, enabling the total digestion of large quantities of dietary lactose. For many people, the source of this dietary lactose tends to come from milk and dairy products.

Lactose intolerance is the most commonly diagnosed adverse reaction to cow's milk among adolescents and adults. I believe that the media attention given to this condition in recent years is what has led to the misconception that humans can't naturally digest milk from other mammals. The main symptoms of lactose intolerance include flatulence, bloating, diarrhoea and abdominal pain which are caused by undigested lactose passing from the small intestine into the large intestine (or colon). The bacteria which are normally present in the large intestine then ferment this undigested lactose. This results in the production of gas which causes the symptoms of flatulence and bloating. Diarrhoea is often caused as a result of more fluid being drawn into the gastrointestinal tract due to the lactose not being absorbed.

There are two ways by which lactose intolerance can be acquired:

1. Primary lactase deficiency/non-persistence

2. Secondary lactase deficiency

Primary lactase deficiency is a genetically inherited decrease in lactase activity, and it often tends to present between the age of 5 and 20 years. It is rare for an individual to experience a total reduction in the activity of this enzyme and more often than not, there is just a partial reduction. This reduction in activity is permanent and cannot be improved by consuming large quantities of lactose-containing foods again.

Secondary lactase deficiency is only a temporary reduction in lactase activity and is often caused as a result of damage to the area of the intestine where the lactase enzyme is produced. There can be a number of causes for this, such as severe gastroenteritis, untreated coeliac disease and inflammatory bowel disease. The symptoms of secondary lactose intolerance normally disappear once the intestinal wall has recovered, which is normally within 2-4 weeks.

The partial loss of lactase activity that occurs after weaning, reportedly affects up to 70% of the world's population. However, the reason why many of us can continue to digest lactose into adulthood, (i.e. ongoing high lactase enzyme activity as we age) is thought to be due to milk and dairy products continuing to be a part of the adult diet as a result of dairy farming. Dairy farming tends to be most common in Northern European countries where the climate is more suited to dairy farming and as a result, it is thought that only 5% of the population suffer any degree of lactose maldigestion. In countries where milk and dairy products are not traditionally consumed as part of the adult diet, many individuals have low levels of the lactase enzyme, meaning they may be unable to digest lactose well and are likely to experience the symptoms associated with lactose intolerance.

In principle, the symptoms of lactose intolerance are dose-dependent given that there is usually some lactase activity still present. This essentially means that some individuals may be able to tolerate small amounts of lactose even after a diagnosis of lactose intolerance, but ingestion of larger amounts might result in more pronounced symptoms. By carefully experimenting, it is possible to find out the amount of lactose that can be tolerated without any adverse symptoms. There are now many products available which have a reduced lactose content which can be useful for individuals who can tolerate only small amounts of lactose in their diets. There are also commercial lactase enzyme preparations, both in a liquid form which can be added to dairy products before consumption, or in tablet form which can be taken before consuming a food product that contains lactose.

Lactose intolerance can be tested in a few ways. It can either be done by having an intestinal biopsy or by two non-invasive procedures: checking blood glucose levels after ingestion of a lactose source or via hydrogen breath testing. Both of these non-invasive measures do have their shortfalls, but if you are concerned that you may be lactose intolerant, go and see your doctor to arrange some testing to rule out that or any other medical condition.

If digestive problems are believed to be as a result of lactose intolerance, individuals can also try a diet without milk and dairy products and other lactose-containing foods for 2-3 weeks to see if their symptoms improve. When milk is reintroduced again and the symptoms reappear, lactose intolerance is likely. Given that this can mean a reduction or exclusion of milk and dairy products from the diet, which we know are important sources of many essential nutrients (e.g. protein, calcium, and other vitamins and minerals), it is important to not avoid them without good reason or without the guidance of a Dietitian. This can help to ensure that you are aware of all the foods which are likely to contain lactose and what to watch out for on food labels (lactose is widely used as an ingredient in many foods), as well as to ensure that your diet is nutritionally adequate.

ARE HORMONES OR ANTIBIOTICS ADDED TO COW'S MILK?

The concerns regarding the ingestion of hormones from milk and milk products has come from the news that in some countries, hormones may be added to the diet of dairy cows to enhance their milk production. In the UK, hormones are not added to milk or to the diet of dairy cows. The milk sold in the UK and in European countries is rigorously tested for traces of antibiotics under European law to ensure that food is safe for consumption. Cows receiving antibiotics are milked separately from the rest of the herd. This milk is then discarded and does not enter the food supply.

To summarise this somewhat complex topic, humans can digest milk and dairy products as long as there is the presence of the lactase enzyme. Milk in the UK and European countries is rigorously tested to ensure there is no presence of hormones or antibiotics and that it is fit for human consumption.

Disclaimer

Discussing dairy, particularly on social media, often brings with it a lot of differences in opinion. I feel that it is important to say here that I am neither pro-dairy nor anti-dairy. I'm not here to share my personal opinions on this, and I don't get paid by any dairy companies to promote any dairy products. I am simply sharing the evidence and science behind dairy products so that you can make an informed decision for your own food and health choices.

The situation in the US is slightly different. Often, certain hormones have been approved for using with livestock, such as dairy cows. The FDA monitors and regulates what is allowed based on current research. If you are curious about the milk you are consuming, it's always good to check out fda.gov.

'CLEAN' EATING

How many of us are familiar with the social media hashtag #cleaneating? This term has been popping up everywhere in the last few years, a common term used by many individuals behind health and fitness social media accounts to describe their eating pattern or dietary choices.

The term implies that a food can either be considered as 'clean' or 'dirty', suggesting that there are certain foods which are 'good' and 'bad' for us and that we 'should' or 'shouldn't' be eating. The term 'clean' is often used to describe foods which are fresh, natural and unprocessed, (e.g. fruit and vegetables etc.) and the term 'dirty' is usually used for those which are highly refined or processed, containing lots of fat, sugar and salt (e.g. chocolate and crisps, etc.). Associating these words with certain foods can often lead to unnecessary restriction, often bringing with it feelings of fear and anxiety about what we should and shouldn't be eating. This, in turn, can result in some individuals developing an unhealthy and obsessive relationship with food. There are many who try to eat 'clean' and don't realise that they can be eliminating important food groups unnecessarily, resulting in the elimination of vital nutrients. Not only that, trying so hard to avoid food viewed as 'dirty', can often have an impact on an individual's social life and their enjoyment of eating out or participating in special occasions or events.

Now don't get me wrong, I don't believe there's anything wrong with trying to share a bit of food inspiration on social media. My worry is that there are some people who don't realise the impact they have on others with the language they use to describe food. This is a topic I talk about frequently on my social media accounts. It's so important for us all to be careful about where we get our nutritional information. Follow trustworthy, evidence-based professionals who encourage balance and inspire you to be the healthiest, happiest and fittest version of yourself.

Nutritionally, it is obvious that there are foods which are considered better for your health than others. However, I truly believe that every food has a place in our diet and any good Dietitian and Nutritionist will tell you the same. There are foods that exist purely to make us feel good because they taste that good. These, I like to refer to as 'soul foods'. Yes, it is important for both your health and energy levels to focus on eating and enjoying nourishing, whole foods, the majority of the time but in turn, you should never feel guilty for allowing yourself the enjoyment of indulgent foods, every now and then.

SUPERFOODS WHICH CURE DISEASE AND HELP WITH WEIGHT LOSS

The term 'superfood' is often used to describe foods which are claimed to have health 'superpowers'. It's a misleading term which should be interpreted with caution.

The short answer is that there is really no such thing as a superfood and we should be concentrating on our diet as a whole in order to stay healthy, not just focusing on the consumption of one food in particular.

Many foods described in this way make bold claims, suggesting they can prevent or even cure a range of illnesses due to a certain nutrient or anti-oxidant present. There's a long list of foods that have been given 'superfood' status over the years – kale, blueberries, beetroot, goji berries, green tea, pomegranates, quinoa, wheat grass and garlic, to name but a few. The term is, in many instances, plastered all over the packaging, often with celebrity endorsement, encouraging you to buy it (and many times with a hefty price tag!). However, the research into this area is largely weak and inconclusive, with no evidence to suggest that one food in particular has a major impact on health or disease prevention. One of the reasons why is because we all have complex diets and it is difficult to separate the effects of one particular food or compound from all of the other foods we consume. This means that many of the studies behind the superfood claims have limitations and we are very rarely told about the limitations when they are reported in the media.

Due to these very deceptive health claims, the EU has now banned the use of the word 'superfood' on any product packaging unless the claim is backed up by convincing research. As a result, a number of well-known brands have been forced to drop this description. However, food manufacturers still try to get around this by using elusive statements describing the health benefits to be gained on their packaging in order to encourage you to buy them. What I would remind you of here once again, is that if it sounds too good to be true, it probably is. Don't believe everything you see or hear on the media.

When it comes to keeping healthy, it's best not to concentrate on any one food in the hope that it will work miracles for you. To optimise your health, the current advice continues to be to eat a well-balanced diet containing a wide variety of foods to make sure you get all the nutrients your body needs for it to function at its best. You also need to limit your intake of alcohol and foods which are highly processed and high in fat, sugar and salt, and aim to maintain a healthy weight and to stay physically active.

Food & Gut Health

The human digestive system consists of the gastrointestinal tract (i.e. the tract through which food is passed after we eat it) plus the accessory organs of digestion (e.g. liver, pancreas etc.). Digestion is a complex process. It is responsible for breaking down food so the nutrients contained therein can be absorbed and used by the body, removing waste products, as well as playing an important role in our immune system. Having a healthy digestive system is absolutely vital for maintaining our overall health and well-being.

Lots of research is going on at the moment on the subject of our digestive system and how different lifestyle factors can have an impact on its function. We already know that disease, stress, medication and diet can all have an impact on our digestive system which, in turn, can cause many distressing symptoms, such as bloating, flatulence, abdominal pain, diarrhoea, and constipation. So it's really important to do what we can to manage the lifestyle factors that we have some control over, in order to optimise and maintain our digestive/gut health.

To encourage good gut health, we should all follow a healthy, balanced diet by including a wide variety of food as already mentioned in this book. That being said, it can also be useful to be aware of the other diet and lifestyle factors which can have an impact on the functioning of our digestive system too. To make it easy for you, I have highlighted some of the main factors over the next few pages and have put them into two different groups: food and lifestyle factors which are thought to be good for our gut health (i.e. Gut Friendly), and those which have been found to have a negative influence on our gut health (Gut Deterring).

GUT FRIENDLY FACTORS

MEALTIMES

One of the biggest things we can control to optimise our gut health is the food we eat and the patterns in which we do this. Adopting a regular meal pattern and making sure you don't skip meals is one of my top tips to help support a healthy digestive system. This means your digestive system isn't getting food erratically all the time, which can help stabilise and regulate digestion. Think about it. The same applies to most humans. Most of us like to have a bit of structure in our lives, as it reduces unexpected stress. The same applies to your digestive system.

Another important thing is to take enough time to eat your food, limiting distractions as much as possible. This means cell phones down, computers and TVs off. Sit down, chew your food well and take your time.

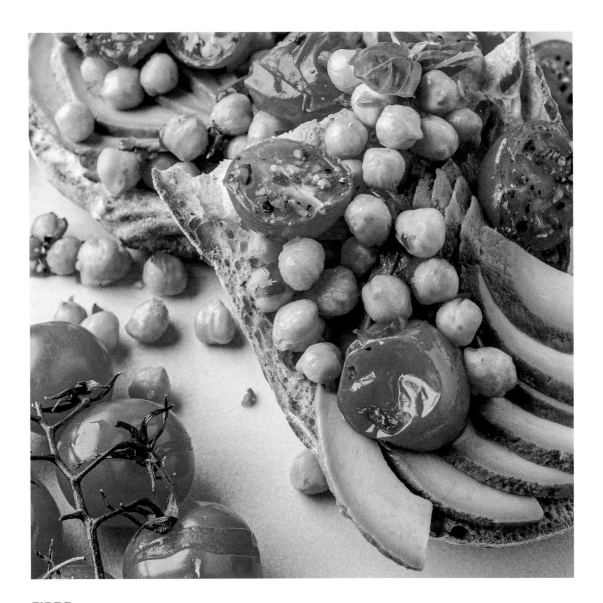

FIBRE

Fibre is required for the normal functioning of the gut; bulking out and speeding up our stools, fuelling our gut bacteria, and playing an important role in immunity and the digestion of nutrients. Fibre was explained in more depth in the Carbohydrate section of the book. I mentioned that there are two main types of fibre and that a combination of both should be included in our diet: soluble fibre and insoluble fibre. Both are required to optimise our gut health, as well as provide lots of other health benefits too.

Remember, don't increase your fibre intake all at once. Build it up gradually, and depending on your digestive symptoms, if you feel that you need any further guidance on this, please seek advice from a Dietitian.

PREBIOTICS AND PROBIOTICS

Our gut contains lots of good bacteria which play an important role in our defence against bugs and toxins, as well as in the digestion of nutrients. It's a common misunderstanding that bacteria are a bad thing but in the case of gut bacteria, they are a good thing. There are so many different types of bacteria found in our gut, and it's essential for us to encourage a thriving gut microbiome by consuming a healthy diet which provides both prebiotics and probiotics. So what's the difference?

Prebiotics are non-digestible food ingredients that only our gut bacteria can feed on. Including these in our diet can consequently encourage the good bacteria in our gut to grow. Not only that, but they are also thought to prevent the growth of potentially harmful bacteria in our gut. The main types of prebiotics in our diet come from a type of carbohydrate known as fructo-oligosaccharides. Food sources are plant-based sources of soluble fibre such as onions, garlic, asparagus, leeks, artichokes, wheat, soybean, oats, chicory and bananas. In the UK, we don't tend to eat large quantities of these foods, so sometimes manufacturers add foods which have prebiotic properties to their food products, such as yoghurt, breakfast cereals and cheese products. It is thought that including prebiotics regularly in the diet can also result in a lot of potential health benefits including, improving the function of the immune system, reducing blood cholesterol levels, helping with mineral absorption, and helping to relieve constipation and the symptoms of irritable bowel syndrome. However, more evidence is needed to strengthen the evidence associated with these claims.

Probiotics, sometimes referred to as 'good bacteria', are live microorganisms which can be found in food products. They are capable of moving through our digestive system and reaching our large intestine (colon) where they are then thought to improve our gut heath by increasing the amount of good bacteria that is already found there. The types of bacteria present in the large intestine can influence our health both positively and negatively, so it is thought that if we are able to increase the levels of 'good bacteria', there will be a more positive influence on our health. Research into probiotics has found some positive effects, suggesting that they may be useful in cases of antibiotic-related diarrhoea, in treating constipation, optimising our immune system and improving some of the symptoms associated with irritable bowel syndrome. Although further research is needed in order to clarify these results, no adverse effects of taking probiotics have been found to date. Although the benefits of probiotics may require further study, their intake is considered as safe. It is worth mentioning here, however, that those who have an impaired immune system may wish to seek specific advice from a doctor or Dietitian prior to taking probiotics. Many probiotic bacterial strains are now added to foods such as dairy products, sauerkraut, kimchi, kefir, and kombucha. Other pickled ingredients are usually good sources, too. Probiotics are also available as supplements in the form of capsules or sachets.

HYDRATION

The importance of staying hydrated was discussed in depth earlier. It has a huge impact on our general health and well-being, but also has a direct impact on our bowel habits. Be sure to drink plenty of fluids every day to meet your requirements, especially water or other non-caffeinated drinks.

RELAXATION

Many people don't relate stress and anxiety to their gut health, but they are strongly connected. The example I often give, which I'm sure many of us can relate to, is the upset stomach we can often experience when we are nervous about something. This can either have an impact on our appetite or make us run to the toilet more often than usual. The gut has its own network of nerves which make up part of our nervous system. Our nervous system takes signals from the brain, which means that psychological factors, such as stress and anxiety, can directly influence the muscle contractions in our gut causing some of the symptoms mentioned previously. This connection between the brain and the gut is known as the Brain–Gut Axis, and its influence on our general health and well-being should not be underestimated. Being good at recognising and managing our stress levels can therefore be really effective in easing symptoms.

So many of us lead very busy, hectic lives and being able to find the time to relax can be something of a struggle. Nevertheless, stress management techniques can be quite simple, it's sometimes just about recognising when we need to use them. Some of my favourites ways to relieve stress are:

» Create time for relaxation.

I appreciate that this can be difficult for many of us, but I really can't emphasise the importance of it. It can be as simple as taking a bath, reading a book or going for a walk.

» Try relaxation therapies.

At the end of 2016 I was given the opportunity to attend one of the free 8-week Mindfulness courses that was being offered through my NHS work. I'll admit, I was sceptical about it at first, but it was actually one of the best things I have ever done. I'm someone who overthinks things and worries unnecessarily about things. Attending this course has really helped me manage this. Some of the things I learned were how to be present in the moment (how many of us have brains with too many tabs open at the one time?), how to deal with unpleasant events in our lives, mindful movement and different types of meditation practice. I know many people have their minds made up about whether this would work for them, so did I, but I would honestly encourage anyone who struggles with stress, to find a trial course and try it with an open mind.

» Take part in regular exercise.

Usually when exercise is suggested as a means of stress management, people imagine having to do tough, gruelling workouts. That's not the case (though of course it can work for some!). For many it can be as simple as going for a walk, going for a swim, leisurely cycling, or taking part in a yoga class.

There is so much research that has been done on physical activity and the impact it has on our heath, not just on the prevention of disease, but also on mood and stress management.

» Prioritise your sleep.

It's scary how many of us don't get enough sleep every night. I was also once guilty of this, thinking that foregoing sleep would mean having more time to get things done so I could be more productive.

That really couldn't be further from the truth. Sleep is so important, not only for our overall general health, but it can also play a vital role in stress management. Getting enough sleep means that we not only function better the following day, but we're far more mentally and physically prepared to deal with any stress that may come our way.

PHYSICAL ACTIVITY AND EXERCISE

Physical activity was mentioned as being something that can have a positive impact on our stress levels, which in turn can improve our gut heath. However, physical activity and exercise can also play an important role in helping us to achieve and maintain good bowel habits. This is because regular physical activity can help encourage regular bowel movements as it helps to stimulate the intestines to work, leading to easier bowel movements. The exercise does not have to be strenuous either. It can be as simple as walking or doing daily living activities, like housework.

GUT DETERRING FACTORS

CAFFEINE

Caffeine is a stimulant found in tea, coffee, hot chocolate, cola and some other soft drinks. It stimulates your bowel by causing it to contract and relax more, which can increase the frequency of your bowel movements. A few cups of tea or coffee a day are usually okay for most people but everyone should be aware that taking too much caffeine can also cause unpleasant symptoms such as abdominal pain, looser bowel movements, as well as have a negative impact on our sleep.

ALCOHOL

We all know that drinking too much alcohol isn't good for our overall general health and well-being, but alcohol also has a direct effect on our gut health, too. Alcohol is known to have a laxative effect which can worsen symptoms of diarrhoea and there is also more research being done on the effects alcohol can have on our gut microbiome.

SOFT DRINKS

Soft drinks are full of bubbles and fizz which can cause a build-up of air in the stomach. This can also cause bloating, excess wind and abdominal pain. Not only that, but soft drinks often tend to be full of artificial sweeteners and caffeine, which can have a laxative effect on our digestive system.

ARTIFICIAL SWEETENERS

The most common artificial sweetener is known as Sorbitol. It is known to be poorly absorbed and induces a laxative effect when it enters the large intestine (colon), which can result in symptoms of bloating and diarrhoea as well. It is found in many products such as low-sugar sweets and drinks, mints and chewing gum. Other types of common artificial sweeteners are Mannitol and Xylitol, which can have a similar effect on the gut. Always check product labels before you buy.

PROCESSED/HIGH-FAT FOODS

Foods which are highly processed or refined tend to contain high levels of fat and sugar and low amounts of fibre. Fibre, as we already know, has many gut health benefits, meaning we should eat more fibrous foods whenever possible. Processed foods also tend to contain a lot of other artificial substances such as additives and preservatives, which our bodies aren't naturally equipped to process.

Foods which are high in fat can be harder for our bodies to digest and as a result, can cause stomach pain and heartburn, in addition to diarrhoea. This includes foods such as fast foods, pies, cheese, pizza, creamy sauces, crisps, chocolate, cake and biscuits, and fatty meats such as burgers and sausages.

We should therefore choose more wholesome, fresh foods whenever possible.

IRRITABLE BOWEL SYNDROME

While we are on the topic of food and digestive health, I'd like to mention a condition which affects many people known as Irritable Bowel Syndrome (IBS). IBS is a medical term used to describe a variety of different gut symptoms, such as bloating, abdominal pain or discomfort, passage of mucus or disordered bowel movements (e.g. diarrhoea, constipation with straining, bowel urgency, and incomplete evacuation). It is a common, relapsing, and often life-long condition, which mainly affects people aged between 20 and 30 years. IBS is diagnosed by the exclusion of other intestinal conditions such as inflammatory bowel disease and coeliac disease; therefore, there is no specific diagnostic criteria. This can make it challenging to diagnose, and often results in many people self-diagnosing the condition. Self-diagnosing can be dangerous if other, more serious bowel conditions are not ruled out first. With the correct professional diagnosis, you can be given the most appropriate treatment and advice from Doctors and Dietitians to best help manage your symptoms.

At some point or other, most of us are likely to experience times when we are affected by some of the intestinal symptoms I've mentioned. This can be due to a number of reasons (as discussed earlier in this chapter); however, it's important that if you have any ongoing troublesome gut problems that you discuss them with your GP to rule out any other alternative cause.

Food & Mood

The food we eat can have an influence, both on our mood and on how we feel. The opposite of this is also true, that how we feel can have an impact on the food we choose to eat. Understanding this relationship can be important and can be useful to help people understand their eating patterns and explain why they feel the way they do.

Eating well can help to provide all the nutrients your body needs to function at its best by improving our digestion and optimising our energy levels. We discussed the main nutrients earlier in this book and it is clear that many of them have an influence on important brain and bodily functions. However, there are some specific nutrients which are believed to have a greater influence on our mood than others.

TRYPTOPHAN

Serotonin is a neurotransmitter (or chemical messenger) in the brain which plays an important role on our mood. The release of Serotonin from our brains is known to improve our mood and influence how we feel. Serotonin is made partly with the help of an essential amino acid called Tryptophan, which we must obtain through our diets. Serotonin is often referred to as our 'happy hormone' because higher levels of this neurotransmitter have been associated with improved mood levels. As a result, low levels of Tryptophan have been linked to possibly causing low mood and depression, due to its role in the making of Serotonin. For this reason, we should ensure that we include sources of this essential amino acid in our diet regularly. Meat sources tend to contain all the essential amino acids; however Tryptophan can also be found in foods such as dairy products, nuts, bananas and eggs.

CARBOHYDRATES

As we know already, glucose obtained from the breakdown of carbohydrates is needed to provide both the body and the brain with energy. It is known that the brain actually uses about 20% of the body's overall energy supply, meaning that it is important that we provide enough energy to the brain for it to function at its best. We also know that by consuming a regular intake of complex carbohydrates, we can keep our blood sugar levels within the recommended ranges, preventing spikes and dips in our energy levels. Not consuming enough carbohydrates can make us feel weak, tired, and subsequently reduces our levels of concentration. That being said, although it is important to ensure we provide our body with regular sources of carbohydrate, consuming carbohydrates in excess will not boost your brain power or concentration to a greater degree.

As well as improving levels of concentration, carbohydrate-based foods are also thought to help more of the 'happy hormone' serotonin to travel to the brain, suggesting that carbohydrate-based foods can also improve our mood. Understanding this can also help to explain 'comfort eating' which is when we eat sweeter foods to help boost our mood. More research into this area is needed, as there is not currently enough evidence to show that eating lots of tryptophan or eating a lot of carbohydrates can really support mood improvement in humans. However, it does suggest that at least we need to make sure that we are eating enough of these foods.

Sticking with this idea of 'comfort eating', it's also necessary to discuss the reward phenomenon, whereby we treat certain foods as being a reward because they make us feel happy after we've had a bad day, (e.g. eating chocolate or ice cream etc.). Although such foods may boost our serotonin levels slightly, the boost in our mood is thought to be more likely to be related to the cultural idea that such foods are considered as reward and comfort foods, rather than this being related to any significant physiological effects particular to the actual food itself.

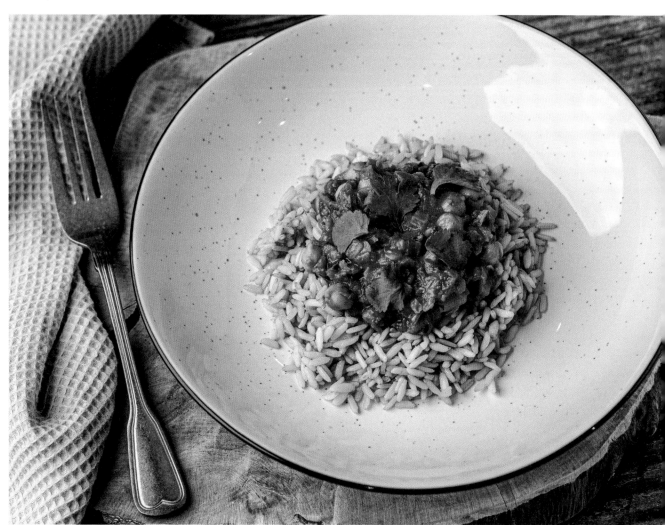

VITAMINS & MINERALS

Not eating a well-balanced diet containing all the vital vitamins and minerals we need, can often have a negative impact on our energy levels, our mood and our brain function. Some of the common vitamins and minerals which can affect our mood are:

» **B vitamins**
B vitamins help us to produce energy from the food we eat, meaning if we don't consume enough of them, we can feel tired, lethargic and low in mood.

» **Iron**
Low iron levels mean our bodies have less haemoglobin, a component of the blood which circulates oxygen throughout our bodies. This can leave us feeling weak, tired and lethargic as well.

» **Folate**
Low Folate levels have been found to be associated with an increased likelihood of feeling depressed.

» **Selenium**
Low levels of Selenium may increase the incidence of feeling depressed and other negative mood states.

OMEGA-3 FATS

Currently, there is substantial research being conducted which is looking into the consumption of Omega-3 fats and the effect that they have on our brain functions and our moods. More evidence is needed to confirm this relationship but we do know that we should be including them regularly in our diet, given that they already have many other confirmed health benefits. The relationship to our brain function and mood, if confirmed, will just be an added bonus. Omega-3 fats can be found in oily fish, flaxseed, walnuts, chia seeds and some fortified products.

WATER

We already know that not drinking enough water can be bad for our health for a number of reasons but with regards to mood, being dehydrated can cause headaches, fatigue, lack of concentration and subsequently, a low mood.

CAFFEINE

Caffeine – the stimulant often found in coffee, cola and energy drinks, can temporarily improve our alertness and counter the effects of fatigue. Caffeine is often considered a 'drug' and too much of it, particularly in individuals who are not used it, may cause adverse effects, such as irritability and headaches. Those who become dependent on many caffeine 'fixes' in their day-to-day lives often find that these symptoms also occur during the withdrawal of caffeine from their diets.

It is clear that feeling good comes from consuming foods and drinks that provide adequate amounts of energy and all the different nutrients we need. Again, it all comes back to consuming a varied, well-balanced diet without an excess of refined/processed foods, alcohol and caffeine. This should guarantee that we are providing our bodies with a good supply of nutrients which are needed for both good health and for boosting our mood.

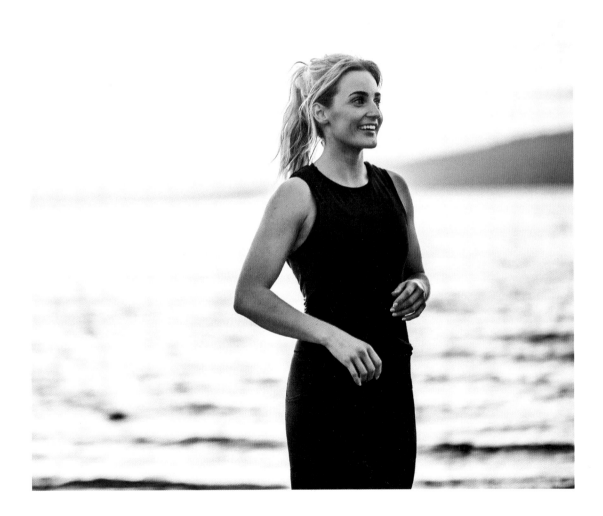

Food & Skin Health

How we can improve the condition of our skin is something I am asked regularly and was often a question I wanted the answer to for myself as well.

During my teenage years and during periods of stress (e.g. exams, etc.), my skin would, and at times still can, break out in spots/pimples, which had a negative impact on my mood. Not only that, but I often felt my skin was dry and somewhat tired-looking and I couldn't understand why. Even so, people who know me would say that my skin was never that bad. But for someone who was not used to wearing make-up, it really annoyed me and as a result, my self-confidence was low. I then started trying to keep my blemishes covered up and ended up using so many skin-care products to try to improve my complexion, which in the end, only worsened the problem.

It's well known that hormones can have a major impact on the condition of our skin and as a result, spots and acne are common for many people during different stages of their lives, (e.g. puberty, menopause and periods of stress). I recognised that hormones were the major cause of my own skin problems at the time; however, with my constant desire to do what I could to achieve better skin, and also with my interest in nutrition starting to develop, I began to look into how my dietary intake could also play a role in my skin health. During my teenage years, particularly when I was at high school and had more freedom in the food choices I made, my diet was pretty unhealthy. I ate out with friends at local cafés and fast food places and snacked on lots of highly processed foods which were high in fat and sugar. As for hydration, I know I definitely didn't drink enough water for how active I was. After taking the time to learn more about nutrition and skin, it hit home to me that my diet was likely playing a major part in the condition of my skin. The food we eat affects every organ in our body and naturally people tend to forget that the skin is an organ as well. A good skin care routine is important, of course, but I am a firm believer that many of us need to focus more on what we are putting into our bodies, and therefore into our skin, rather than just what we are applying to the surface of it.

When first discussing the connection between diet and skin health with my clients, I like to begin by looking at what they should be including in their diets, rather than what they should be taking out of them. Hopefully, it is reassuring to know that no food has to be completely avoided, but we also need to keep in mind that there is no one specific food that can work magic and give you a healthy glow. You'll have noticed that I've said this before, but it all comes down to eating a healthy, well-balanced diet containing a wide variety of foods. This will help to ensure that you are including food sources that provide the right nutrients which are known to be beneficial for our skin, including Omega-3, vitamins A, C and E, vitamins B2, B3 and B6 and the minerals zinc and selenium. Refer back to the Macronutrient and Micronutrient Section of the book for more information on the function of these nutrients and what food sources you can find them in.

Although that's a lot of nutrients to think about when it comes to skin health, the good news is that a varied and well-balanced diet which includes food sources from the 5 main food groups will provide all these nutrients without you having to worry about each specific one. Evidence from lots of studies have shown that by following healthy eating guidelines, your body will get all the vital nutrients it needs to support skin health and anti-ageing.

HYDRATION

The typical thing that you hear when it comes to skin health is to make sure that you stay hydrated – and it's so true. The skin is made up of water to a great degree which not only helps to prevent fluid loss, but also works to hydrate and moisturise the skin cells. So, staying well-hydrated is very important for keeping the skin moisturised and supple, as well as for improving the appearance of fine lines and wrinkles by maintaining the skins' elasticity.

SUPPLEMENTATION – IS IT NECESSARY?

A food-first approach is always the best way to give our skin and our bodies the nutrients they need. If you manage to eat a well-balanced diet that provides you with sources of all the different nutrients you need, then you shouldn't need to take a supplement. Although we know that certain nutrients are beneficial for skin health, it doesn't mean that consuming more of them is better for us. Anything in excess is never a good thing. On that note however, if you are concerned that you may not be getting all the essential nutrients from your food intake, you should speak to your GP and see if you need to be referred to a Dietitian.

OTHER LIFESTYLE FACTORS THAT CAN AFFECT OUR SKIN HEALTH

GETTING ACTIVE

Exercising regularly and choosing activities that get the heart working a little more can help improve blood flow to the skin's surface which can help improve your skin's natural glow.

DITCHING THE CIGARETTES

Smoking is known to increase the skin's ageing process. This is because the toxins found in smoke prevent the skin from producing a normal amount of collagen. A lack of collagen is associated with the development of wrinkles.

Milk and Acne?

This is something else I am asked about all too often. Many share the belief that milk is the cause of their acne; however, there is currently no convincing evidence to back up this claim.

What I always say is that everyone is different. One food can agree with one person and not with another. Milk and dairy products are an important source of nutrients in the diet, providing the body with protein and lots of vitamins and minerals. Before making any unnecessary dietary exclusions, you need to take a look at your diet and lifestyle first, and then make sure there is nothing else that you can do to optimise your skin health. Not only that, but you should keep in mind that more often than not, the cause of acne may often be related to hormonal factors which we have no control over.

If you still believe that it is milk and dairy that is causing your skin problems and you wish to exclude these from your diet, it's important to make sure you take fortified dairy free alternatives to provide you with the nutrients you will be missing out on. If you feel you need help doing this, it's always recommended that you seek advice from a Dietitian.

RESTING AND RELAXING

Sleep is thought to play an important role in our skin health, because this is the time when the body can effectively get to work and renew and repair cells and tissues, etc. Making sure we get plenty of sleep can help keep our skin looking young and, at the same time, prevent it from looking tired.

Research has also shown that too much stress can have a negative impact on our skin health, too. Make sure you take some 'Me Time' during stressful periods or consider learning some stress management techniques, such as mindfulness and meditation.

AVOIDING UV RADIATION EXPOSURE

We all know that too much time in the sun is the primary cause of skin ageing due to the exposure to the UV radiation in sunlight. Ultraviolet light damages the collagen and elastin in our skin which we need to keep our skin smooth and supple. Too much sun can cause wrinkles, dry, rough skin, and more seriously, can increase the risk of skin cancer. Never allow your skin to burn and always use sun cream with a sun protection factor of at least 15.

HAVING A GOOD SKIN CARE ROUTINE

Many skincare products claim to have the power to prevent or reverse the signs of aging skin, but unfortunately, most of these claims don't have high quality scientific evidence to back them up. However, there are benefits to finding a suitable topical skin care regime that works for your skin type, to cleanse away dirt and moisturise the skin's surface. This not only helps to keep the skin in good condition, it helps to protect it from the environment and also prevents it from drying out.

Plant-Based Diet

Following a plant-based diet has really started to grow in popularity in recent years. It describes a diet which is based on foods which are derived from plants, including fruit and vegetables, whole grains, legumes, nuts and seeds, with just a few or no animal products. However, the phrase 'eating more plant-based' can also describe someone's attempt to reduce the amount of animal products they are consuming.

Some people choose to follow a plant-based diet or eat more plant based for a variety of reasons, some of which include a dislike for the taste and texture of animal-based products, concern about the treatment of animals, health reasons, financial reasons, social pressures, and also as a result of environmental concerns associated with livestock farming.

DIFFERENT PLANT-BASED DIETS

There are many variations of a plant-based diet so here you can find an explanation of some of the more common ones.

Plant-Based Diet Variation	Description
LACTO-OVO VEGETARIANS	Lacto-ovo vegetarians eat dairy foods and eggs but no meat, poultry or seafood.
OVO-VEGETARIANS	Ovo-vegetarians include eggs in their diet but avoid all other animal foods, including dairy.
VEGANS	Vegans don't eat any animal products at all, including honey, dairy and eggs. This requires very careful planning and checking of food labelling as many ready-made products can contain animal ingredients even if they don't contain any obvious meat or dairy.
PESCETARIANS	Pescetarians eat fish and/or shellfish but do not eat meat.
FLEXITARIANS	Flexitarians is the name given to people who are semi-vegetarian, meaning that they may occasionally eat meat or poultry.

Given that meat and dairy products provide a vast amount of nutrients to the body, it's really important to find suitable, alternative food sources for these nutrients if you decide to eat more plant-based. However, if plant-based diets are well planned, they can support healthy living at any age. The term I would like to stress here is 'well-planned'. I hear far too often of situations where people decide to go more plant based – often excluding complete food groups, which usually supply a rich source of nutrients in their diet – and they make this dietary change with no consideration for the nutritional implications this can have, if done without some very specific knowledge and careful planning. It is also common for some people to decide to follow a plant-based diet for the sole purpose of weight loss, believing that the removal of meat and dairy products will help them shed the pounds. Done correctly, a plant-based diet which is well planned and low in foods containing saturated fat can help with weight management and may help to reduce the risk of health conditions such as type 2 diabetes, cardiovascular disease and some types of cancer. This is because high consumption of red or processed meat can provide high levels of saturated fat and have been associated with higher risk of certain health conditions. However, I believe that eating a plant-based diet shouldn't be done solely for the purpose of weight loss, but instead should be done with the focus on improving health by helping to reduce the intake of red and processed meat. As a result of poor planning, I personally know many cases in which people have actually gained weight by changing to a plant-based diet. This is often because they over-compensate for the removal of certain foods they usually include in their diet by consuming larger portions of food from other food groups (e.g. large portions of carbohydrates and snack foods such as crisps/chips, chocolate and biscuits/cookies etc., which can still be included, depending on the particular plant-based diet being followed).

Plant-based diets that focus on the inclusion of a wide variety of plant-based foods such as wholegrains, fruit and vegetables, beans, nuts and seeds, can provide all the nutrients needed for good health in an affordable, delicious and nutritious manner. However, if you are minimising or avoiding all animal-derived foods, there are a few nutrients that you need to pay particular attention to for good health:

PROTEIN

Animal products are a rich source of protein which is required for the growth and repair of body tissues, and for providing essential amino acids. Plant-based sources include lentils, beans, chickpeas, seeds, nuts, nut butters and tofu. Depending on what foods you wish to include in your diet, eggs and dairy are also great sources of protein. Meat substitutes can also provide a source of protein, however some of these products are highly processed, often containing high amounts of fat, sugar and salt, so should therefore be enjoyed in moderation. Those following a plant-based diet should also ensure that they are obtaining all the essential amino acids required for health by eating a wide variety of plant-based protein sources. Check out the section on Protein in the Nutrients chapter of this book for more information on this.

CALCIUM

Calcium is an essential mineral required for bone health. Milk and dairy products are the richest source of calcium in the diet, so if you choose to avoid them, it's really important that you get calcium from other sources. This can be either from fortified plant-based dairy alternatives or natural plant-based sources such as tofu, leafy green vegetables, dried fruit, some nuts and seeds, etc. Check out the section on Bone Health for more information on this important mineral, and to make sure you're meeting your calcium requirements.

OMEGA-3 FATS

These unsaturated fats can provide an array of health benefits and the richest sources of them are known to be oily fish. If you do not include fish in your diet, there are plant-based sources of Omega 3 fats which you should consume regularly to be sure your body reaps the nutritional benefits of this essential fat. Look at the section on Fat in the Nutrients chapter of this book for more information on this essential nutrient and for suggestions on the plant-based sources in which it can be found.

VITAMIN D

We already know that vitamin D is needed to keep bones, teeth and muscles healthy, and that the main source of this vitamin comes as a result of the skin being exposed to sunlight. There are some animal food sources of vitamin D, including oily fish, meat and eggs, in addition to a few plant-based sources, such as sun-exposed mushrooms and fortified foods, vegetable spreads, and plant-based dairy alternatives. In the UK, most people are thought to obtain enough of this vitamin through sunlight exposure and dietary sources. However, during the winter months, we all need to get vitamin D from our diet because the sun isn't strong enough for the body to produce this itself. Since it's difficult to get enough vitamin D from food alone, everyone should consider taking a daily vitamin D supplement during the autumn and winter months. More information on this topic can be found in the Micronutrient and Bone Health sections of the book. It is also worth noting here that some vitamin D supplements are not suitable for vegans, and special attention must be paid to reading the ingredients on the food labels.

VITAMIN B12

Vitamin B12 has many important functions in the body and an untreated deficiency of this vitamin can cause a number of unpleasant symptoms such as fatigue, anaemia and nerve damage. Our richest source of this vitamin is animal products, and when following a plant-based diet, the only sources which can be relied on are fortified foods and supplements. Some examples of fortified foods include some breakfast cereals, non-dairy milks, soya milk, soya yoghurts and soya desserts, as well as yeast extracts. If you are avoiding animal produce, to make sure you are getting enough vitamin B12, you should aim to consume fortified foods at least twice a day or a vitamin B12 supplement may be needed. If you have concerns as to whether you are getting enough of this essential vitamin, I recommend speaking to your GP.

They can assess your levels, decide on whether a supplement is required, and also determine whether or not you should be seeing a Dietitian who can help make sure you are optimising your dietary intake as much as possible.

IRON

The richest and best-absorbed source of iron comes from animal-based products such as red meat and eggs. Plant sources include dried fruits, whole grains, pulses/legumes, nuts and seeds, green leafy vegetables and fortified plant-based products (e.g. some bread and breakfast cereals). The form of iron found in plant-based foods is not absorbed in the body as efficiently as the form found in animal sources. If you are avoiding animal products in order to help improve your iron absorption from plant-based sources, you should aim to take them alongside a source of food rich in vitamin C, such as citrus fruits, strawberries, green leafy vegetables and bell peppers.

IODINE

Iodine is an essential mineral which the body needs in moderation to support a number of important bodily functions, such as the normal functioning of the thyroid gland, the maintenance of our body's metabolic rate, body temperature regulation and for brain and central nervous system development. The major sources of iodine in our diet are from fish and milk and dairy products. The iodine content of plant foods differs greatly and depends highly on the iodine content of the soil in which the food was grown. Foods which are grown closer to the ocean tend to be higher in iodine. Where soils are iodine-deficient, iodised salt and seaweed can provide iodine. This mineral is only needed in moderation and since the iodine content of seaweed can also vary (and is sometimes too high), the recommendation is not to consume sea-grown vegetables more than once a week, especially during pregnancy. Iodised salt is not widely available in the UK but can be found in some supermarkets. However, since it is recommended that we limit our salt intake for health reasons, you shouldn't rely on iodised table salt as a means of increasing your iodine intake (see Salt Intake & Health). Individuals who avoid both meat and dairy products are consequently at risk of developing an iodine deficiency. A supplement containing iodine can help meet your needs if you do not consume sufficient iodine-rich foods, however, you should speak to your GP before taking a supplement to make sure you don't exceed the recommended amount. Seaweed or kelp supplements are also not recommended and should not be used. This is because the amount of iodine in these products can vary considerably from the value claimed on the label and can provide excessive quantities, which can cause negative health effects. When in doubt, speak to your GP and ask to be referred to a Dietitian for more guidance and advice.

ZINC

Zinc is an important mineral which plays a vital role in many bodily functions. It is involved in: producing lean body tissue and hormones, the processing of carbohydrates, protein and fat contained in the food we eat, helping to maintain normal hair, skin and nails, assisting with wound healing and supporting normal fertility and reproduction. Zinc is best absorbed from animal sources. This is because plant-based sources contain a mineral known as phytic acid which reduces zinc absorption. The effects of phytic acid can be reduced by soaking plant-based sources and cooking the food first before it's eaten. Plant-based sources include fermented soya (e.g. tempeh and miso), beans, wholegrains, nuts, seeds and some fortified breakfast cereals.

SELENIUM

Selenium is a trace element which helps to maintain the function of the immune system, prevents damage to the body's cells, and is needed for the production of thyroid hormones. Our richest sources again, tend to be animal products, but there are many plant-based sources of this mineral, too. Brazil nuts are thought to be one of the best plant-based sources providing the recommended daily allowance in the consumption of just two nuts! Other plant-based sources include grains, seeds and other nuts.

SUSTAINABLE EATING

Food is known to be the single strongest key to optimising both human health and environmental sustainability on Earth. Environmental sustainability is now one of the major reasons that many people choose to follow a completely plant-based diet or consume a more plant-based diet. This is due to the concerns about the environmental damage being caused as a result of livestock farming. Meat and dairy farming are thought to be the leading contributors to greenhouse gas emissions and globally, food production is known to be threatening our climate's stability as well as the resilience of our ecosystem. Not only that, but food production is also thought to constitute the single largest cause of environmental degradation.

There is more and more research being done to look into this area with emerging evidence suggesting that reducing animal-based food consumption and eating a more plant-based diet can be beneficial not only for our own health and well-being, but also for the health of our planet.

Improving Your Relationship With Food

Knowledge is power, and improving your understanding of nutrition is one of the first steps towards improving your relationship with food. From the evidence-based nutrition advice I have provided you with so far, you now have the power to apply this advice and reap the benefits of what a healthy, balanced diet can do for your mind, body and soul.

Although it's great to have all this amazing nutritional knowledge, it's also really important to understand and appreciate why we sometimes choose the foods we do, as well as for us all to look a little deeper into and seek to understand the relationship we have with our bodies. Doing this can really help identify problems with our own individual eating patterns so we that we can acknowledge and deal with them, as well as learn to practice some self-love and to value and respect our bodies just the way they are.

COMFORT EATING

Comfort or emotional eating is often used to describe the action of turning to food for comfort and escape during times of low moods or stress. Doing this can temporarily improve our mood so we briefly feel comforted and soothed, but this is usually short-lived because comfort eating does not resolve what was the cause of the issue in the first place.

Don't get me wrong, enjoying food as a reward or a 'pick-me-up' from time to time is a totally normal and natural part of life. However, when it is used regularly as the only strategy of dealing with troublesome emotions, it can often lead to more serious problems of disordered eating. Eating disorders are very serious health conditions needing special medical attention and support. They are a whole separate topic entirely and deserve a book of their own.

Emotional hunger is very different from physical hunger. It tends to come on suddenly and brings with it the feeling that it needs to be satisfied immediately. It can lead to cravings for specific foods, which, more often than not, are foods which are higher in fat and sugar. Even though we may eat this desired food in a large quantity, they often leave us feeling unsatisfied despite our stomachs being full. And finally, one of the biggest problematic associations with this form of eating is that it can often bring feelings of guilt, shame, lack of control and powerlessness.

There is still a lot to learn about the causes of comfort and emotional eating and the more serious eating disorders that often are associated with it. This is because there is usually not just one main cause or trigger that causes emotional eating, and it is likely to be as a result of many different factors which play havoc with our coping mechanisms.

WHAT ARE THE SIGNS OF COMFORT/EMOTIONAL EATING?

There are a number of signs of emotional eating, which can generally be divided into 3 main categories: behavioural, physical and psychological.

» **Behavioural**
Behavioural signs include, eating in secret, social withdrawal and isolation, hiding food packaging and buying lots of extra food.

» **Physical**
Physical signs can include symptoms such as bloating, stomach pain, nausea, poor skin, weight gain, poor sleep and fatigue.

» **Psychological**
Initially people will experience feelings of comfort and relief when they eat, but this is often followed by feelings of anxiety, depression, guilt, shame and worry.

Comfort and emotional eating often go hand in hand as a coping mechanism. If this becomes an individual's default treatment for coping with their emotional needs and feelings, this often suggests that they have a lack of alternative coping strategies. Building up a bank of coping strategies will better equip us to deal with problems more effectively, rather than turning to food to overcome problems.

One of the first steps is to identify the triggers which cause you to reach for food as a form of comfort and support. This involves creating an awareness of the feelings which have resulted in your eating and understanding and appreciating the feelings that tend to come afterwards.

Was it hunger that made you eat, or was it boredom or stress? Did you feel satisfied and well-fuelled afterwards or did you still feel hungry and experience feelings of guilt and worry, too?

To help identify these triggers, I often encourage keeping a Food & Mood Diary. This can be a really useful tool to help you become more aware of the food you are eating, your feelings at the time, and ultimately help you recognise and identify the root of the problem.

If you feel this is something that could help you, I have included an example of a Food & Mood Diary on the next page. It encourages you to note down the time and location of when and where you eat, how hungry and how satisfied you were before and after you ate, and some space for you to write down any feelings you have to help you identify any common themes.

Whatever themes or patterns you manage to identify from using the Food & Mood Diary, don't let them get you down. Acknowledge them and accept them. Identifying some of the likely causes of emotional eating will make you feel proud as you have just taken one giant step forward towards improving your relationship with food.

FOOD & MOOD DIARY

Time	Location	Food and Drink Consumed	Hunger Level	Satisfaction Level	Additional Comments

Enjoying food as a reward from time to time is totally normal. We must always remember that, especially when it comes to days when we didn't eat as well as we would have liked. That's completely normal, too. No one is perfect. No one gets it right 100% of the time. Sadly, I think social media is mostly to blame for creating the idea that we need to get it right all the time. The huge surge in the number of health and fitness social media accounts over the last few years has resulted in many people sharing their healthy eating inspirations. They're full of colourful, mouth-watering photos, which begs the question – where are all the "real-life" photos of people eating pizza and chocolate? Remember, the majority of people on social media only want to share with the world the times they feel they look good and so they post things that society should consider as 'the ideal'. I understand this. People fear being judged so if they share themselves being anything other than perfect, people might not look up to them anymore. Don't get me wrong, there is nothing wrong with a bit of healthy eating inspiration, but I worry about the lack of balance that we see on the internet, and the healthy eating tips being shared by those who are not qualified. Be careful who you follow on social media, who you take nutritional advice from, and always remember, social media accounts very rarely give accurate reflections of a person's whole life. You only see what they want you to see.

I firmly believe that mindset is everything. If you experience a day where you didn't eat well, just accept it and move on. Put "your positive pants on" and try to do better the next day. If you do your best to create a mindset like this, whereby you both accept and believe in yourself and you encourage your mental and emotional attitude towards focusing on more of the positive aspect of situations, you can really influence your thoughts and behaviour on a daily basis. This doesn't always mean simply smiling and looking cheerful. It refers to an overall perspective on life and describes a tendency to focus on all that is good in life. The more you can mentality anticipate happiness, health and success, the more you can strengthen your belief that you can overcome any obstacle or difficulty.

My Tips

For Being More Positive

1. **Be optimistic.**
   Be willing to make an effort and take a chance, instead of assuming your efforts won't pay off.

2. **Demonstrate acceptance.**
   Acknowledge that things don't always turn out the way how you want them to, but learn from your mistakes.

3. **Show resilience.**
   Bounce back after experiencing adversity, disappointment, and failure instead of giving up.

4. **Be grateful.**
   Continuously appreciate the good things in your life.

5. **Be mindful.**
   Dedicate your mind to conscious awareness and enhance your ability to focus. Consider attending a mindfulness course or learning meditation.

6. **Show integrity.**
   Be honest, righteous, and straightforward. Doing anything else just over-complicates life.

MINDFUL EATING

Mindful eating, sometimes also referred to as intuitive eating, describes the process of raising awareness to what we actually eat. This involves being fully present in the moment, taking in every colour, taste and texture of the food we eat to fully appreciate the sensations, thoughts and emotions that come along with it. This should be done without any judgement on your part to help you appreciate and enjoy your food more.

How many of us have been in the situation where we're standing up while we eat or eating on the go because eating can seem to be a chore sometimes on the days when we have about a million and one things to do? How often are these the days when we just seem to inhale our food, clearing our plates before we even realise it, and still not even feeling satisfied with what we have just eaten?

Mindful eating is here to help with this and the interest in this technique has grown greatly in popularity in recent years to help us become more in tune with our bodies. The idea behind this is that by being more aware of what we are actually eating, we can create the potential for choosing healthier options, recognising when we are full, which in turn, can have a positive influence on weight management.

I personally learned a lot more about mindful eating when I took part in a Mindfulness course a few years ago. It sparked my interest in this somewhat new and interesting area, and I truly believe the concept has the potential to work wonders for so many of us.

Essentially, we want to limit distractions while we eat and make sure we are fully present in the moment. This can be done in a number of ways, including:

» Reducing distractions – phones, TVs and other technology should be put away at mealtimes

» Sitting at a table while eating, rather than on the sofa

» No eating on the go or when standing up

» Chewing your food slowly and taking your time

» Recognising when you are eating as a result of some emotion

» Forgetting the idea that eating well doesn't count at the weekend, just because you have been good all week

» Not eating food for the simple reason that it's just because it's there, right in front of you

By considering the above scenarios, this will hopefully get you thinking about the reasons why you sometimes eat the way you do. Being able to recognise these reasons and accept them without any judgement on your part can really help you on your way to eating more intuitively with your body. It can also enhance the process of nourishing your body and improve your overall enjoyment of food.

HOW TO BE A MINDFUL EATER

1. Mindful Hunger

When you feel hungry, become aware of your body, and think about exactly what your body is telling you. Spend a couple of moments noticing the sensations that give you that message of hunger. By listening to your body more, your body will be able to tell you if it is actually hungry and what it is hungry for. You should be doing this without judgement and accepting your feelings for what they are. By doing this, you can learn to accept and understand the real feelings of hunger, rather than just automatically reaching for food when it might not be exactly what you need.

2. Mindful Food Choice

When choosing what to eat, you need to take your time and be fully aware of exactly what's on offer. Think about the difference between the foods which are on offer, what they're made of, how they are prepared and how they smell, etc. Notice and accept that the choice of food is yours, and what thoughts or feelings arise from each option, without trying to change these thoughts or feelings.

Doing this can help you to become more aware of the choices you make, encouraging you to make more informed choices that nourish you— whether that's by eating something fresh or wholesome, or something more indulgent that is good for the soul.

3. Mindful Food Prep

It's also important for you to be mindful as you prepare the food you are about to eat. That might be as you peel, chop and cook something, or simply when you open a food product package. Become more aware of the textures, sounds, smells and what it looks like as your food is placed in front of you. Remember, we eat with our eyes and our noses, too. Paying attention to our food helps prepare the body for digestion, which can make our digestive system and our appetite signals work better too.

4. Mindful Eating

Start by having a good look at what you're about to eat. Appreciate the textures, shapes and colours, then, be aware of any smells and sounds that come from it. When you take a mouthful, fully appreciate the taste, textures and temperature of the food and how it feels in your mouth. Take your time to chew it and savour every single bite. This allows you to appreciate the food you eat and also allows the body to respond appropriately by creating feelings of enjoyment from the meal, easing the digestive processes and signalling when you're full.

5. Mindful Fullness

After you have finished what you're eating, keep that body awareness. A good way to do this is to focus on your breathing. Appreciate the different feelings you are experiencing. This can include feelings of satisfaction (or dissatisfaction!), any movement within your body, or any lingering tastes. Becoming more aware of feelings and sensations after you have finished eating can allow your body to comfortably return to a resting state, which in turn, can improve your digestion. Not only that, but increasing your awareness and appreciation for natural feelings of fullness can also help prevent habitual overeating.

Enjoy Everything in Moderation

This is one of the most common phrases that you hear people saying when the topic of nutrition comes up. Everyone talks about how we should find 'balance' in our lives, but I can appreciate that many people get frustrated by this, as they don't know what balance actually means for them. The difficulty with this is, is that 'balance' looks different for everyone. What works for one person may not work for another, and it's all about finding a balance that works for you, and only you. Having 'balance' can be applied to anything we do in life, not just our nutritional intake. We all hear about trying to achieve that work: life balance and the importance of this is well understood. To encompass everything, I believe that achieving 'balance' is finding a place in your life where you are eating, moving, working and living in a way that makes you the happiest and healthiest version of yourself.

Remember what I have already said. No one gets it right 100% of the time and that's totally okay. Life throws things at us all the time, and this alone can challenge the equilibrium of our balance. It's about being able to adapt to challenges and accepting that it's okay that we don't always get it perfect. Sometimes it's just about protecting our energy at the present moment, and then continually trying to get back to that place of happiness in whatever way we can.

When it comes to achieving balance with regards to our nutritional intake, this is where I really believe in the power of education. Educating yourself on how to eat healthy will provide you with the power on how to nourish your body but will also give you the freedom to relax when it comes to enjoying the more indulgent food that we all know and love. I have already mentioned my love for the term 'Soul Foods' and feel it's such a good way for us to remember that the food we eat shouldn't just be thought of as fuel for the body. Food should not only be thought of as a key to nourishing our bodies to keep us healthy, but can also be considered at times as a way of nourishing our souls by providing us with a source of delicious happiness that we can enjoy with family and friends.

Placing unnecessary restrictions on your nutritional intake usually throws moderation out the window and often results in binge eating. Binge eating usually occurs because we have missed the food we have been excluding, causing us to over-compensate when we choose to eat it again, often leaving us with feelings of shame and guilt. This is not balance. Believe it or not, including the odd indulgent food in our diets every now and then is actually good for us. Allowing yourself this freedom by not restricting certain foods will reduce the likelihood of obsessing over them and then binge eating them.

By achieving this balance, you will provide your mind, body and soul with nourishment which can lead you to a place of body confidence and content.

WARNING: If you believe or recognise that you are suffering from an eating disorder or any other form of disordered eating, I would encourage you to seek professional help. You can do this by going to see your GP in the first instance, who will refer you to the appropriate health professionals who can help you. You can also choose to see private health professionals if you prefer. Don't go through this alone. Finding happiness and balance really is achievable, and there is so much help and support available to help you get there.

Being Your Own Motivation

People ask me all the time, how do I stay motivated to eat well and exercise so often? My honest answer is that I don't. I don't have a magic solution. There are so many days when I have zero motivation, and most of the time, I just get up and do it anyway, because the rewards are usually always worth it. Motivation is never going to be a constant thing. It comes and goes, and it is rarely there when you want it or need it most. The key is to create sustainable habits and become disciplined, to help support you when your motivation is low. Habit and discipline can teach you how to become accountable for your health and well-being and can help set you up for life.

Motivation is usually what gets us started, but how many of us can relate to trying to be super healthy, planning to make a whole bunch of lifestyle changes, trying to make all the changes at once, then failing to keep the momentum going? Sound familiar? This all comes down to us setting our expectations too high and then trying to change too much at once. That being the case, we need to make sure that our end goals are realistic and achievable, so we don't have unrealistic expectations which can set us up for failure and disappointment. This is why it's so important for us to set suitable behavioural goals to help us to achieve success.

There is a common goal-setting theory or set of principles that I like to use with clients who are trying to make any kind of dietary or lifestyle change. It's called S.M.A.R.T., which is an acronym for a set of goal-setting criteria. Using the S.M.A.R.T. principles when setting our own goals can not only help identify suitable end goals, but it also encourages us to identify appropriate and realistic steps on how best to achieve them.

The theory suggests that for a goal to be motivating, it should be:

Specific
Measurable
Achievable
Relevant
Timely

For a goal to make a difference in the time set to achieve it, it needs to be as far-reaching as possible. Goals need to be specific so that you can have direction and focus on how to reach it. Rather than setting vague goals such as 'I am going to eat more healthily', you need to be more specific and identify those areas of change within your own diet which will help you do that. A more suitable S.M.A.R.T. goal would be 'I will increase the portions of fruit and vegetables I eat from 1 to 3 portions every day'. This goal is far more achievable, as it gives us precise direction, fitting in with the S.M.A.R.T. criteria.

Another important thing to think about here is the number of goals you set. Only two or three specific, achievable and realistic goals should be set at any one time, identifying the small steps you need to take on how to get there. This will increase your likelihood of success, help you to stay motivated, and allow you to continue building on your goals. In the long-term, focusing on just a few goals at a time will also help you to gradually develop your own sustainable habits which you can maintain for the rest of your life.

To motivate you to achieve your goals, implementing rewards can also be really useful to help keep you going. Rewards should never be food-based as this only creates the idea of food restriction and increases the likelihood of using food to provide comfort/emotional support. Instead, suitable rewards could be: doing an enjoyable leisure time activity (e.g. going for a massage or to a spa), being with your favourite people (e.g. going to the cinema or out for a meal at your favourite restaurant with people you love), buying small things that you want (e.g. a new pair of shoes or new active wear) or doing something else you find relaxing or fun. Make sure you congratulate yourself regularly on every effort and achievement, no matter how big or small. You have to keep cheering yourself on as no one else can do it for you 100% of the time. This can really help you to stay consistent and can have such a positive influence on your feelings of self-worth, self-esteem and self-belief in your own ability to change.

My Tips

For setting goals

Something I always encourage people to do once they have set their goals is to write them down someplace where they are visible. This could be on your cell phone, in a diary or journal or on a white board in your home. This should also be someplace where it can easily be seen on a daily basis to give you a constant reminder and motivational boost to keep going.

The Dark Side of Social Media

There is more pressure on us to be healthy, now more than ever before, and I personally feel that it's at the point where many people are competing with one another to be the best. This could be with family, friends or even with other people on social media. Social media is one of our biggest influencers today, and I believe there can be so many positive benefits with using it. However, with the surge in the number of health and well-being social media accounts there are on the internet, there has also been an increase in the number of people who are not qualified to offer nutritional advice, yet they still do. Please remember that just because someone has lots of followers and looks 'good' in their photos, doesn't mean they actually know what they're talking about when it comes to nutrition and fitness. Just because a celebrity or 'social media influencer' decides to exclude something from their diet, is trying out some new diet product, or following a new diet trend, doesn't mean that you should be doing it, too. It's also important to remember that many celebs and social media influencers are asked by companies to market their products for them through the internet to increase these companies' sales. This is usually for money – and often quite a lot of it. Not only that, but the products that they promote are often bad for our health and can encourage a negative relationship with food and our own bodies. At the time of writing this book, there has been a lot of attention on this topic and I hope that one day celebs and influencers will be banned from promoting diet products. Individuals who do this are doing it with a total disregard for the actual health and well-being of the many vulnerable people they seek to influence.

The same freedom is open to you when someone tells you that they have decided to go vegetarian or vegan. This doesn't mean that you have to do this, too. You need to experiment with your own nutritional intake to see what makes you feel good and what makes you thrive. This is what I hope this book will allow you to do. I want it to really empower you to make your own decisions on your own dietary and lifestyle choices, making you feel confident because you know that you have the scientific evidence behind your choices. Don't compare yourself with anyone else. Go on your own journey to nourishment, doing it in your own way and in your own time.

Seeing Changes

I mentioned back at the beginning of the book that one of the most liberating things that I have ever done was throwing away my bathroom scales, and I encourage you to do the same. Don't get me wrong, weight can be a useful measurement at times (e.g. to help a Dietitian to work out estimated nutritional requirements, or a pharmacist to work out how much of medication you may need), but the majority of the time, all it does is demonstrate your relationship with gravity. Weighing yourself too often only causes fear, distress and anxiety. Many people use their body weight to determine the success of their lifestyle changes, but many people are unaware that body weight actually changes on a daily basis due to a number of factors, such as shifts in our fluids balance, and whether we have been to the toilet. Many individuals often lose motivation and get very disheartened if they step on the scales and see that their weight has increased after they have started exercising and have made dietary changes. However, they don't often realise that they are actually building their muscle tissue with exercise, and muscle tissue weighs more than body fat. Weighing yourself on your bathroom scales does not give a true reflection of your body composition.

Instead of weighing yourself so often, you should congratulate yourself on having made these dietary and lifestyle changes and focus on the wider health benefits that these changes are bringing you.

The human body and each of our individual personalities are all wonderful. Why would we let a number define our self-worth and dictate our happiness and who we are as a person?

When you embark on your own health journey, I encourage you to track your efforts in other ways. This could be taking progress photos or noticing how you feel in your clothes. I also encourage you to focus on the small gains which likely have a much bigger impact than you realise. This could be by enjoying better energy levels, feeling stronger, sleeping better, seeing improvements in your skin and your digestive system. Focusing on health improvements such as these can be far more motivating and rewarding.

Sleep

We all know how lousy we can sometimes feel if we haven't slept long enough or if our sleep was disturbed in some way. This can leave us feeling drained and exhausted, both physically and mentally. However, the health cost of sleepless nights is more than just being in a bad mood or having a lack of focus the day after. It has been found that having poor sleep on a regular basis puts you at higher risk of experiencing other more serious health conditions, including obesity, heart disease and diabetes, which in turn, can have a negative influence on our overall life expectancy

As I mentioned before, I used to forego sleep to be more productive, and it took me a while to realise that this was actually having the total opposite effect. Prioritising my sleep has made such a big difference to me in so many areas of my life, including improving my work productivity, enhancing my mood, increasing my energy and concentration levels, and improving the quality and success of my workouts.

HOW MUCH SLEEP DO WE ACTUALLY NEED?

The answer to this is also different for everyone. Most of us need around 8 hours of good-quality sleep a night to function properly, but some people may need more and some people may need less. The important thing is to find out just how much sleep works best for you and then try every night to reach your own sleep goals. A good indicator of whether you're getting enough sleep is to notice if you routinely wake up feeling tired and then spend the rest of the day looking for a chance to nap or look forward to going to bed again. If that's the case, you are probably not getting enough sleep.

WHY IS SLEEP SO IMPORTANT?

SLEEP CAN AFFECT OUR WEIGHT

Many studies have shown that not getting enough sleep on a regular basis can play a major role in weight gain. This is thought to be the result of sleep both influencing certain hormone levels in our body, which can influence our appetite, and reducing our energy levels to stay motivated to exercise due to feeling tired and lethargic. If we are sleep deprived, we can have decreased levels of a hormone called Leptin and increased levels of a hormone called Ghrelin. Both of these hormones can influence our body weight by reducing our ability to feel full and by stimulating our appetite. How many of you have ever noticed that after a poor night's sleep we tend to eat bigger portion sizes and can often crave food that will give us that quick boost of energy (e.g. chocolate and sweets)?

SLEEP BOOSTS OUR MOOD

I'm sure many of us have experienced the feeling of being grumpy and irritable the day after just one poor night's sleep. Chronic poor sleep has, therefore, been related to even more serious mood disorders, such as depression and anxiety.

SLEEP ENHANCES OUR PERFORMANCE

This can affect any aspect of our life – work, sex, or sports performance. Prioritising sleep is so important for boosting energy and concentration levels, improving the libido, and enhancing strength and endurance levels.

SLEEP HELPS PREVENT HEALTH PROBLEMS

More and more research shows that getting enough sleep can reduce the risk of developing a number of serious health conditions such as Type 2 Diabetes and Heart Disease. The processes behind this are complex, but it may be the result of an increased risk of obesity related to sleep-deprivation, or possibly due to more specific drivers such as an increased heart rate, higher blood pressure or sleep deprivation having a direct effect on certain hormone levels. Sleep deprivation has also been linked to potentially causing reduced fertility in both men and women.

SLEEP BOOSTS OUR IMMUNE SYSTEM

Sleep deprivation has been shown to have a negative impact on the functioning of the immune system. This can make it difficult for the body to fight off infections and therefore increases the risk of coming down with an illness, cold or flu or becoming unwell in general.

My Tips

To Improve Sleep

If you're someone who doesn't get enough sleep, here are my top sleep tips to help you get a more a restful night.

Tips to Improve Sleep	Why Does it Help?
Bedtime Routine	Have you ever noticed that you tend to feel full of energy and tired at the same times every day? This is because of your circadian rhythm – a 24-hour internal clock that runs in the background of your brain. It cycles between sleepiness and alertness at regular intervals and helps tell your body when it's time to wake up or go to sleep. You can help regulate this clock by giving yourself a set time to go to bed and get up every morning, doing the same at the weekends. Work back from what time you usually need to get up, allowing yourself an adequate number of hours to sleep, and this will give you what should be your regular bedtime. Avoiding bright lights in the evening, and exposing yourself to sunlight in the morning, can also help regulate your circadian rhythm. Find a bedtime routine that works for you and stick with it.
Unplug and Wind Down	Having a relaxing bedtime ritual is so important for helping to prepare the body for sleep. This means using no technology and staying away from bright lights just before you go to sleep.

Your own ritual could be having a warm bath, doing relaxation stretches or gentle yoga, reading a book, listening to relaxing music or audiobooks, or organising a 'To Do List' for the next day to help organise your thoughts and reduce stress. Doing this can also help you to separate yourself from your day-time activities which can often cause stress or excitement, helping you to fall asleep easier and improving your sleep quality. |
| Create a Sleep-Friendly Environment | Your sleeping environment plays an important role in the quality of your sleep. Keep your bedroom just for sleep and intimacy, and nothing else. No work should be done in your bedroom, and you should avoid unnecessary bright lights like that from TVs, phones, and alarm clocks. For optimal sleeping, you should make sure your bedroom is dark, quiet, tidy and cool. |

>>

Physical Activity	Getting your body moving every day is a great way to improve your sleep. Exercise at any time of day is fine, but I would suggest avoiding vigorous exercise just before going to bed.
Naps	If you have trouble sleeping, it's best to avoid naps, especially in the afternoon. It's all about creating that regular sleeping pattern and routine. Power napping may help you get through the day if you're feeling exhausted. I would recommend setting an alarm for 20 minutes maximum as anything longer can result in you going into a deeper sleep, making you wake up feeling worse. However, if you are struggling to fall asleep at bedtime, eliminating any day-time naps could help.
Food	Eating big, heavy meals before bed can cause discomfort from indigestion that can make it harder to get to sleep. Try to have your last main meal of the day about 2-3 hours before bedtime and enjoy a light snack about 30-60 minutes before bed if you feel you need it. Sugary foods before bed should be avoided, too. They can give you a blood sugar spike and a boost of energy, which could make it difficult for you to get to sleep.
	Also avoid alcohol and cigarettes in the evening. They act as a stimulant and can make it difficult for you to get to sleep and can also affect your sleep quality.
Caffeine	We all know caffeine has its benefits, helping us to feel more alert and reducing feelings of fatigue. However, caffeine has a long half-life, meaning it takes a long time to get out of our system. Avoid any caffeinated drinks later than 5-6 hours before bedtime. If you're struggling with sleep, try to drink fewer caffeine or energy drinks during the day as a pick-me-up. They may boost your energy and concentration temporarily but can also disrupt your sleep pattern even further in the long run.
Sleep Diary	A Sleep Diary can be a really useful tool to help you wind down before bed by giving you a place to write down your thoughts and clear your head. It can help you track your sleep as well as allow you to see habits and common trends that are either helping or hindering your sleep.

Alcohol

We all know that we should limit the amount of alcohol we consume, both in the short- and the long-term, due to the health implications associated with it. Excessive amounts can be severely toxic and potentially dangerous as a result of the loss of co-ordination, self-control and change in behaviour it causes. In the long-term, excessive alcohol consumption is known to cause very serious health conditions such as liver disease, pancreatitis and some cancers. The risk of developing these illnesses increases with any amount of alcohol we drink on a regular basis. However, if we keep within the recommended limits, we can reduce this risk.

There have been many claims in the media over the years suggesting that drinking certain types of alcohol, particularly red wine, may bring some positive health benefits. However, this evidence is largely inconclusive, and because of this, we should continue to stay within the recommended alcohol limits.

Alcohol isn't classified as an essential nutrient, meaning that we don't need to include it in our dietary intake to support health. However, it does provide the body with a source of energy. Alcohol provides 7 calories per gram and is, therefore, considered calorie-dense in comparison to some of the other macronutrients. This means that our alcohol intake can easily contribute to weight gain. Alcohol is also often referred to as 'empty calories' because apart from providing the body with energy, it provides no other nutritional value. Besides the health problems associated with excessive alcohol consumption, this higher caloric value is another reason that we should all be mindful of our alcohol intake. We should also take into consideration the other ingredients which are in alcoholic drinks, such as sugar, cream and fruit juice, all of which add more calories. Alcohol is also an appetite stimulant. This can result in our eating larger portions of food at mealtimes, late at night and even into the next day until the alcohol is completely out of our system. Not only that, but the food that most people tend to reach for when they are drinking alcohol is food which tends to be high in fat, salt or sugar.

WHAT ARE THE ALCOHOL RECOMMENDATIONS?

In the UK, alcohol is often measured in units, a system which was put in place in the 1980s to help make it easier for people to keep track of their alcohol consumption. However, many people find it difficult to understand and apply.

One unit of pure alcohol is 10ml (1cl) or 8g

The Department of Health (DOH) recommends that we should not regularly drink more than 14 units of alcohol per week, and it is best to spread this evenly over three days or more. This is because there are increased health risks associated with binge drinking.

In the US, the Centers for Disease Control and Prevention recommends a person should consume only moderate amounts of alcohol: up to one drink per day for women and two drinks per day for men.

SO WHAT DOES A UNIT LOOK LIKE?

The number of units of alcohol contained within a drink varies, depending on the alcoholic strength of the drink and the serving size. To help make it easier for you, here are some examples of the units of alcohol found in the standard measures we are more likely to be given in a bar or restaurant.

Alcoholic Drink	No. of Alcohol Units
A small glass (125ml) of ordinary strength wine (12% alcohol by volume)	1.5 units
A standard glass (175ml) of ordinary strength wine (12% alcohol by volume)	2.1 units
A large glass (250ml) of ordinary strength wine (12% alcohol by volume)	3.0 units
A 35ml measure of spirits (40% alcohol by volume)	1.5 units
A pint (568ml) of lower strength lager/beer/cider (3.6% alcohol by volume)	2.0 units
A pint (568ml) of higher strength lager/beer/cider (5.2% alcohol by volume)	3.0 units
A can of lager/beer/cider (440ml) (5.5% alcohol by volume)	2.0 units
A bottle of lager/beer/cider (330ml) (5% alcohol by volume)	1.7 units
Alcopop (A ready-mixed drink that resembles a soft drink but contains alcohol.)	1.5 units

If you're planning a pregnancy or are already pregnant, you are advised to avoid drinking alcohol altogether. This is because alcohol is not only known to reduce the ability to conceive, but it can also damage an unborn baby and may even lead to early miscarriage. If you are breastfeeding, occasional drinking, such as having one or two units once or twice a week, is not harmful to your baby, but drinking any more than this can cause problems. It's also best to avoid drinking alcohol just before breastfeeding because the alcohol can be passed onto the baby in small amounts through the breast milk. If you are ill or suffer from a medical condition such as diabetes, high blood pressure, gastric ulcers or depression, or if you are taking certain medication, you should take extra care or seek medical advice if you wish to consume alcohol. Your GP or pharmacist can help advise you on this.

My advice to anyone who wishes to consume alcohol is to enjoy it in moderation and be mindful of the number of units you are consuming. Alcohol tolerance is different in everyone and it's important to remember that even if you feel you can drink larger amounts without feeling unwell, you are still causing the same damage to your body and putting yourself at the same risk of health problems.

Getting Active

We all know that staying active and exercising regularly is great for our health for a variety of reasons. It not only helps us become fitter and stronger, but it has also been found to help reduce (by up to 50%) the risk of developing a number of major illnesses, such as Type 2 Diabetes, cancer, stroke and heart disease. Staying active is not only known to be beneficial for our physical health, but evidence shows that it can have a positive impact on our mental health, too. Physical activity can boost our self-esteem, lift our mood, improve our energy levels and the quality of our sleep, reduce our stress levels, and our risk of developing depression, dementia and Alzheimer's disease. Whatever our age, staying active is thought to contribute significantly to leading healthy and happy lives.

The evidence supporting the benefits of exercise is overwhelming. It can be free and gives health benefits immediately, and there is a whole variety of ways we can do it. Ideally, we need to do a mixture of cardiovascular exercise and strength (resistance) based exercise each week to reap the benefits. This can be by walking, jogging, cycling, swimming, boxing, aerobic classes, dancing, playing football or other sports. The list is endless. This is why I truly believe that there is a form of exercise out there for everyone, as there are countless different ways that we can move to stay active.

We should all try to do at least 150 minutes of cardiovascular exercise every week, which involves getting our heartrate up a bit and our lungs working a bit harder, as well as including two strength (resistance) sessions each week, when we work on strengthening our muscles.

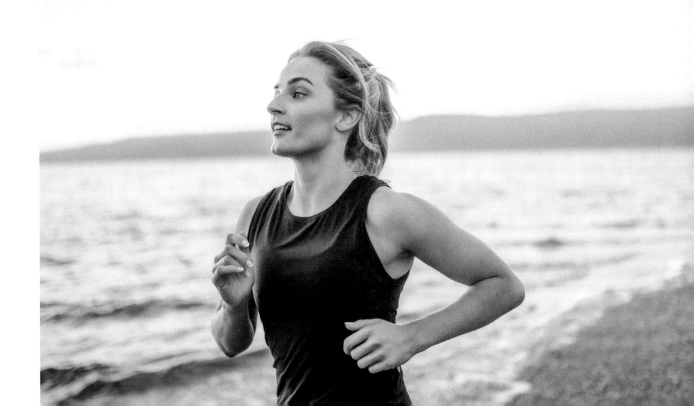

Rewarding Reasons to Exercise

» Exercise because you enjoy it

» Exercise to improve your health

» Exercise because it makes you feel good

» Exercise because it gives you energy

» Exercise because you want to become fitter

» Exercise because you want to become stronger

» Exercise because you want to improve your flexibility and mobility

» Exercise to meet new people

» Exercise because you want to try something new and learn a new skill

» Exercise because you want to challenge yourself and gain a sense of achievement

» Exercise to improve your mood

» Exercise to boost your self-esteem and improve your body confidence

Cardiovascular exercise can be classified into two main groups; aerobic exercise or anaerobic exercise. Aerobic exercise simply means exercising 'with oxygen' and anaerobic exercise simply means 'without oxygen'.

Aerobic exercise uses the presence of oxygen to breakdown carbohydrates and fat to give us energy. This usually involves steady-state cardio exercise where we are moving at a low-moderate intensity, and can last a long period of time (e.g. brisk walking, swimming, running, cycling).

Anaerobic exercise is short-lasting, high-intensity exercise, where the body's demand for oxygen exceeds the oxygen supply which is available. This means the body must use another metabolic pathway which doesn't require oxygen in order to provide the body with energy to complete the exercise. This type of high-intensity exercise is only sustainable for a maximum of about 2 minutes, but it allows us to get energy to our muscles fast to carry out movement or exercise (e.g. sprinting 100m, lifting heavy weights or doing high intensity interval training).

Both types of cardiovascular training have their advantages and have been proven to bring a number of health benefits, including lowering the risk of cardiovascular disease and other chronic diseases such as Type 2 Diabetes, as well as improving blood pressure and cholesterol levels, while, at the same time, encouraging body fat loss.

Strength (resistance) training is a type of exercise which uses a form of resistance to cause your muscles to contract. This resistance can come from simply using your own body weight or by adding in weights such as barbells, dumbbells, kettlebells, resistance bands or the resistance machines you see in gyms. Doing regular strength training encourages our muscles to change and adapt (otherwise known as 'training adaptation') to build their strength and size. This type of training can encourage us to get leaner and stronger by building our muscle mass and encouraging body fat loss. Not only that, but it can also improve bone density, joint flexibility and can help improve our balance.

Many people like to split up their cardiovascular and strength training over the week, allowing for a few rest days each week in between, to allow time to rest and recover. What you do for exercise and how you do it, is entirely up to you. The main thing is that you find a form of exercise you love, which fits easily into your lifestyle.

Despite the benefits of exercise being well known, so many people today continue to lead very sedentary lives. Not only that, but many individuals who do exercise do it for all the wrong reasons, treating it as a chore and as something they have to do for the sole purpose of losing weight. This attitude is something I am so passionate to change and is one of the main reasons why I decided to become a Personal Trainer. I want people to find a form of exercise they actually love and to exercise for other more rewarding reasons, rather than just for weight loss.

Exercising just to lose weight is very rarely an enjoyable experience, and the motivation to continue to exercise can easily fade away. Not only that, but measuring your progress just by weighing yourself alone isn't a good idea, as measuring our body weight does not determine the differences in body composition – see the chapter on Seeing Changes for more information on this.

If you are able to find a form of exercise that you love for at least one or more of the reasons listed, you are far more likely to keep doing it, and changes in your body composition (i.e. fat loss and muscle gain) will likely come as a result of regularity and consistency. One thing I often suggest to people if they are struggling to find the motivation to start exercising, or are worried about trying out something new, is to think about doing it with a friend! This can really improve your motivation both before and during a workout, it can make you far less likely to stop exercising and can even make it really fun, too.

If you don't know where to start when it comes to exercising, or you have an injury that you feel is stopping you, I highly encourage you to think about investing in a Personal Trainer. This can often be the best money you'll ever spend when it comes to getting active and staying active. A good Personal Trainer should be able to assess your abilities, train you, educate you, motivate and inspire you to find your love of keeping active.

At the end of the book, I have also provided you with lots of fun workouts to help inspire you too! There are workouts suitable for all levels of fitness – beginning, intermediate and advanced – allowing you to choose the level that's right for you. Not only that, but there are lots of fun training methods to choose from to help keep your workouts fun, varied and challenging!

Nutrition for Fitness

If you are someone who exercises regularly or takes part in competitive sport, you have the potential to adapt your nutritional intake to maximise your training sessions, optimise your body composition (e.g. build muscle), and ultimately enhance your performance.

For those clients I see for sports nutrition advice, whether that be recreational or elite athletes, the main thing I always stress to them is that they need to concentrate on getting the basics of nutrition right first by consuming a diet which contains food sources from each of the 5 main food groups. The way I often explain this is by stressing that they can't expect to make adaptations to their dietary intake to optimise their performance if they are not eating well for their health in the first place. If they master the basics, only then can they focus on tweaking their dietary intake further in order to enhance their performance.

As a Sports Dietitian, when completing a nutritional assessment on an athlete, a whole range of factors that could be influencing their nutritional intake have to be considered. We must look at the athlete's life as a whole, considering things like the athlete's medical history, their work and training schedules, their body composition, their food preferences, their nutritional requirements in relation to their sport, their current nutritional intake, any practical challenges for optimising their nutritional intake, their goals, and much more. After we complete a full nutritional assessment, we then discuss and agree on appropriate goals to help achieve the athlete's desired outcome. Their progress is reviewed and adapted regularly, in order to increase the athlete's chance of success.

If an athlete is managing to get the basics right with regards to their nutritional intake, further nutritional adaptations can then be made to help optimise their sporting performance. Some of the main things a Sports Dietitian will focus on are; ensuring that the athlete is well fuelled for their sport, and that they consume appropriate quantities of each macronutrient, as well as focusing on what and when the athlete should be eating around their training sessions or competition. For highly trained athletes, there is a fine balance between training hard enough to achieve maximal training results and avoiding the illness and injury risk associated with a high volume of training. Nutrition plays an important role in this. Athletes must ensure that they are well-fuelled and consuming a well-balanced diet that contains all the right nutrients to meet their needs, to help prevent injury and optimise the function of their immune system, ultimately preventing illness. The importance of enhancing an athlete's nutritional intake should not be underestimated and can play a pivotal role in optimising their sporting performance.

ENERGY INTAKE

Every individual, whether an athlete or not, has varying energy requirements on a daily basis. Your energy requirements can fluctuate even more if you exercise often, especially if you are involved in a periodised training programme. It's important to ensure that you are consuming enough food each day to maintain your health and maximise your training outcomes. Not consuming enough energy through your food intake can result in a number of issues, such as; loss of muscle mass, menstrual dysfunction, hormonal disturbances, sub-optimal bone density, fatigue, increased risk of injury and illness, impaired training adaptation and a prolonged recovery process. This cluster of physiological complications caused by an insufficient energy intake is often referred to as Relative Energy Deficiency in Sport (RED-S). If you are experiencing symptoms like these, it's really important that you do not ignore them, and you should seek professional advice and support as soon as possible through your GP and an accredited Sports Dietitian.

On the days you train, it is likely that you will need to consume more energy, through inclusion of a higher amount of macronutrients in your diet. This will allow you to fuel your training sessions appropriately. On rest days, when you are less physically active, it is likely that you will not need the same volume of food as what you would consume on training days. A regular meal pattern should still be followed on rest days, but you may not require as large a portion size, or the same number of additional snacks, given your lower energy requirement.

THE ROLE OF MACRONUTRIENTS IN SPORTS

CARBOHYDRATES

Carbohydrates are the body's preferred source of fuel, therefore it's obvious that this nutrient plays an even more important role when it comes to sport and exercise.

Carbohydrates are vital for achieving the best sporting performance, as exercising muscles rely on carbohydrate as their main source of fuel for movement. The amount of carbohydrates you need will depend greatly on your training programme and your dietary goals. As a general rule, the more intense the training programme, the more carbohydrates you will probably need in order to fuel yourself appropriately.

Diets which are low in carbohydrate have been associated with poor energy levels during exercise, the early onset of fatigue, poor concentration, delayed recovery, as well as an increased risk of illness. This is likely due to a lack of essential vitamins known to be important for immune function, which are often obtained from sources of carbohydrates.

The body has a storage form of carbohydrate which can be found in our muscles and liver, otherwise known as glycogen. Glycogen stores are limited, which means they need to be topped up every day through the consumption of carbohydrate foods. This is particularly important if you exercise most days, or if you exercise at a high intensity, as then you are more likely using up your muscle glycogen stores as a source of fuel. The best way to ensure that you are eating enough carbohydrate is to ensure that you have a regular meal pattern every day. Every meal should be based on the Balanced Plate guidelines mentioned previously, making sure you include a source of complex carbohydrates. Additional carbohydrate-based snacks can be included in between meals, if required, to help meet your requirements and ensure you have sufficient energy for your training session.

How much carbohydrate should I be eating to fuel my sport?

Intensity of Exercise	Carbohydrate Target
Light Low intensity or skill-based activities	3-5g per kg body weight
Moderate Moderate exercise programme (e.g. 1 hour of exercise per day)	5-7g per kg body weight
High Endurance programme (e.g. 1-3 hours per day of moderate to high intensity exercise)	6-10g per kg body weight
Very High Extreme commitment (e.g. 4-5 hours per day of moderate to high intensity exercise)	8-12g per kg body weight

The above recommendations are only a general guide. Carbohydrate intakes should be fine-tuned with individual consideration of total energy needs, specific training needs and feedback from training performance.

PROTEIN

Protein is required for building and repairing muscle, and therefore plays an important role in how the body responds to exercise. If we exercise regularly, our dietary intake of protein should be increased to help support our muscles to adapt and recover well from our training sessions. To support this process, current research suggests that our protein intake should be in the range of 1.2g to 2.0g per kg body weight per day, for both strength and endurance-based exercise. Evidence also suggests that better training adaptation is achieved by meeting your daily protein intake goals by spreading your protein intake regularly throughout the day. This is because your muscles are still adapting for at least 24 hours after completion of a training session. This means that it is not only important that you include a protein source following a strenuous exercise session, but also that you include high-quality protein sources at each meal and snack throughout the rest of the day.

FAT

Fat is an essential component of a healthy diet, providing energy, essential fatty acids and fat-soluble vitamins. Dietary fat guidelines for athletes are the same as that for the general population. This means that fat should contribute to no more than 35% of your daily energy intake. Fat intake can be further individualised based on your training level and body composition goals. However, a fat intake which contributes to any less than 20% of your total energy intake is not recommended, as this will likely have a negative impact on your overall health by subsequently limiting your intake of a variety of other essential nutrients.

You should continue to focus on opting for sources of monounsaturated fats and omega-3 fats where possible, and limit your overall intake of saturated fats.

HYDRATION

Although not a macronutrient, we all know that we should be drinking plenty of fluids each day to ensure we are well-hydrated. A good fluid intake is not only important for general health, but it plays a crucial role in optimising exercise performance. Fluid intakes are very individual, and the best way to maintain and monitor your hydration levels is to meet the minimum fluid recommendations (at least!), and increase your fluids accordingly, using the colour of your urine as a good indicator as to whether you are well-hydrated enough.

If you'd like to get more specific about your fluid replacement needs for your sport, doing a routine measurement of pre- and post-exercise body weight (which ideally takes into consideration any urinary losses and the volume of any fluid consumed) can help to estimate sweat loss during exercise. Generally speaking, a loss of 1 kg of body weight represents approximately 1 litre of sweat loss.

For example:

$$\text{Sweat Loss (mL)} = \text{change in body mass (g)} + \text{fluid intake (mL)} - \text{urine losses (g)}$$

However, there can be a limit to the practicality of measuring urine losses and the exact fluid intake during an exercise session or event. Nonetheless, this could be a useful method of determining a more accurate estimation of your fluid replacement needs.

PRE-WORKOUT NUTRITION

The foods you consume before a training session or event play a vital role in your overall athletic performance. Getting it right can ensure your body is well-fuelled and hydrated for the exercise session ahead, improving the quality, intensity and duration of exercise. Not only that, but it can also help you to avoid any digestive upset and prevent you from getting any distracting hunger pangs during the training session.

The three main nutrients which are important to consider for pre-workout are carbohydrates, protein and fluids. Failing to fuel or hydrate your body appropriately before exercising can hinder your performance in a number of ways. It can cause the early onset of fatigue, reduce your speed and endurance ability, reduce your concentration levels (which can result in skill errors) and can also cause gut upset. It's a good idea to experiment with your pre-workout nutrition during your training, trying different foods which contain these important nutrients. This will allow you to identify those foods which work best for you before you take part in any competitive events.

HOW LONG BEFORE EXERCISE SHOULD YOU BE EATING?

There is 'no one size fits all' answer to this question. Generally, most people can tolerate their last main meal between 2 to 4 hours before exercising without any stomach upset. If further fuel is required before exercising, a small, light carbohydrate-based snack can also be consumed 1 to 2 hours before exercising. For most people, it is better for these snacks to also be low in fat, low in fibre, and have a low to moderate protein content. The low fat/low fibre content will allow for easier digestion and consuming some protein will also encourage the building of lean muscle tissue.

Examples of Pre-Workout Light Carbohydrate-Based Snacks

» Fruit Smoothies made with yoghurt/milk

» White bread sandwich with jam

» A small bowl of cereal with milk/yoghurt and fruit

» Small bowl of white pasta with a tomato-based sauce

» Greek yoghurt with fruit

It's also important to be well-hydrated before an exercise session or event. It is usually better to sip on fluid gradually in the hours leading up to the exercise rather than taking in a huge volume at the one time just before you start. This allows your body to use the fluid effectively, preventing stomach upset and the need to urinate soon after you start exercising. What fluid you decide to drink really depends on your own goals. If you are simply trying to make sure that you are well-hydrated for an exercise session, then water or electrolyte drinks can be a good option. If you are unable to eat food before exercise or an event, you might find that you tolerate fluids better. In that case, ideally your fluids should contain a source of carbohydrates to allow you to top up your fuel stores. This is where sports drinks can be helpful.

NUTRITION DURING EXERCISE

Whether you should eat or drink during an exercise session or event depends on a number of factors, such as the intensity and duration of the exercise, and your own body composition goals. Generally speaking, the two main nutrients to focus on during your exercise session or event are carbohydrates and fluids.

It's very challenging to determine the amount of fluid that is appropriate to meet every athlete's fluid needs. Ideally, you should be well-hydrated prior to exercise and topping up with fluid throughout the session, depending on your sweat losses. Evidence so far has suggested that the fluid intake that suits most athletes should typically provide 400-800mls of fluid per hour, although this may need customising, depending on the individual. The ideal fluid to consume during exercise remains very much dependent on your individual goals and the recommendations remain similar to that described for pre-workout fluid intake.

Regarding carbohydrate ingestion, the recommended amounts to consume during exercise varies greatly, depending on your own exercise intensity and duration. The current recommendations are summarised in the following table.

Duration & Intensity of Exercise	Carbohydrate Recommendation
Brief exercise of < 45 minutes duration	Unlikely to need to top up carbohydrate levels during the session, unless pre-workout nutrition has not been optimised. Regarding hydration, small amounts of fluid may be required, depending on sweat loss rates.
High-intensity exercise of approximately 45-75 minutes duration	Evidence suggests that exercise performance can be optimised by consuming small amounts of carbohydrate during the session to top up fuel stores. To ease digestion and to allow for quick absorption of nutrients, sports drinks and sports products can provide a source of easily consumed carbohydrates, as well as top up fluid levels.
Endurance exercise of 1 – 2.5 hours duration	A higher focus on carbohydrate consumption will be required. Evidence currently shows that consuming 30–60 grams of carbohydrate per hour during such events can help to optimise performance. However, the difficulty often lies in the opportunities available to consume food and drink. What can be tolerated during long endurance events is also very variable. Some individuals can tolerate solid carbohydrate foods, others cannot. If solid foods can be tolerated, similar principles apply to the pre-workout carbohydrate recommendations, whereby ideally foods should be carbohydrate-based but be low in fat and fibre to ease digestion.
Ultra-endurance exercise lasting 2.5 – 3 hours duration	Evidence shows that consuming up to 90g of carbohydrate per hour can optimise performance. The way in which these are consumed, either through solid food or fluids, depends on the athlete's personal preference and tolerance. Hydration levels should also be considered, and fluid levels should be topped up regularly throughout the duration of the session.

It is very much a case of trial and error to find a refuelling and rehydration strategy to use during exercise which is both appropriate and suitable for you. It remains important to experiment with this during your training sessions to find the type and amount of food which works best for you, before you take part in a competitive event.

Examples of Carbohydrate Foods Which May Be Suitable During Exercise

» Muesli Bars

» White bread sandwich with jam or honey

» Fruit muffins

» Carbohydrate gels

» Sports energy bars

» Bananas

» Sports Drinks

POST-WORKOUT NUTRITION

The goals of a post-workout nutritional intake should focus on helping the body to recover from the completed exercise session. This involves appropriately refuelling and hydrating the body, supporting the immune system, encouraging the growth and repair of muscle and promoting training adaptation. Training adaptation refers to the process of the body becoming accustomed to the exercise session and the training load.

The main nutrients to be focused on during the immediate recovery period (0-2 hours post exercise) are carbohydrates, protein and fluids.

The same principles apply to replenishing fluid as those which were previously mentioned. The amount required can vary greatly between individuals and should be based on sweat losses and whether the fluid is needed for hydration only, or for also providing a source of fuel.

Examples of Carbohydrate & Protein Foods Which May Be Suitable Post-Workout

» A well-balanced main meal (see the section, Building a Balanced Plate)

» Greek yoghurt and fruit

» Cold meat sandwich

» Bowl of cereal with milk or yoghurt and fruit

» Spaghetti with lean beef bolognaise sauce

» Chicken wrap with lettuce and cheese

» Small tin of tuna on crackers, plus a piece of fruit

» Boiled eggs, plus crackers

» Low-fat cottage cheese

» Protein shake plus a piece of fruit (see more information on supplements in the following section)

Regarding carbohydrate post workout, the main aim is to replenish glycogen stores. This requires an adequate and timely intake of carbohydrate after completion of the exercise session. Ideally, you should consume 1 to 1.2 grams of carbohydrate per kg body weight per hour in the first 4 to 6 hours after exercising. You can decide for yourself what types of food and/or fluid you wish to choose to meet this recommendation.

The current evidence suggests that an early intake of high-quality protein sources in the immediate post-exercise recovery period will provide the necessary amino acids required to build and repair muscle tissue. Not only that, but consumption of adequate protein may also enhance the replenishment of glycogen stores. You should aim to consume at least 0.25 to 0.3 grams of protein per kg of body weight (this equates to approximately 15-25g protein) in the first 0 to 2 hours post-exercise. Your overall daily protein target should be met throughout the rest of the day through regular consumption of protein-rich foods contained in each meal and snack.

I often suggest that athletes should try to eat a main meal post-workout to meet this higher nutrient requirement. If this isn't practical or possible (e.g. depending on your environment or perhaps your tolerance levels to food after exercise), be prepared and pack carbohydrate and protein-based snacks to take with you.

MICRONUTRIENTS

All athletes should consume diets that provide at least the Recommended Dietary Allowance for all micronutrients. This can easily be achieved if you eat a varied and well-balanced diet which meets all your energy needs. (See the Micronutrient in the Nutrition section for more information).

SUPPLEMENTS

An adequate, well-balanced diet will provide all the nutrients and energy you need for your sport or form of exercise. Unfortunately, many people spend a lot of money on sport supplements, thinking that if they exercise, they need these products and that supplements are the key to sporting success or for achieving their desired body composition goals. However, adding supplements to your dietary intake without taking care to get the basics right first means that supplements can often provide very little benefit. Your goal should always be to focus on optimising your basic dietary intake first and making additional dietary changes afterwards.

That being said, there are some supplements which have been shown to be beneficial for performance or to assist in achieving body composition goals, if taken correctly (e.g. caffeine, creatine, beta-alanine, protein supplements, nitrate, sodium bicarbonate). Each of these supplements can provide different advantages but do not come without a risk of side-effects. Not only that, but they are often expensive and may require specific instructions for use. Products should also only be chosen with consideration of the risk of potential contamination from unsafe or illegal chemicals. If you decide to buy a supplement, make sure you always choose products that have been through rigorous testing for banned substances and, it is recommended that you speak to a Sports Dietitian for more advice.

PROTEIN SUPPLEMENTS

One of the most common supplements I am asked about are protein supplements. If you exercise regularly, you will have higher daily protein requirements to support muscle growth and recovery. For most people consuming a well-balanced diet, especially one which includes animal products, these higher protein requirements can usually be met easily via a food first approach which includes protein sources in meals and snacks consumed throughout the day. In this case, exceeding the recommended protein requirements through the addition of a protein supplement offers no additional benefits for the process of building lean muscle tissue and often just provides additional, unnecessary calories. However, if you follow a vegetarian or vegan diet, or do not consume dairy foods, you may have difficulty reaching higher protein requirements if your diet is not well-planned. In this instance, your priority should always be to experiment with new ways of optimising your dietary protein intake first. If reaching this higher protein target continues to be a challenge, then seeking advice from a Sports Dietitian may be the answer for you. Sports Dietitians can help to establish whether the use of a protein supplement is actually necessary and can provide guidance on which supplement would be best to suit your needs.

The only time when protein supplements may otherwise be useful would be for convenience purposes, to provide sufficient protein post-workout. However, the same advice still stands for you to consume your protein needs through food first, whenever possible. Sometimes all it takes is just a little bit of extra planning and preparation so that you have simple protein-based snacks packed in your sports bag ready to eat after your training session, taking protein supplements only if and when it's absolutely necessary.

The field of sports nutrition is vast and complex. The information provided in this chapter only scratches the surface, providing you with some of the basic advice from the current evidence in this area. If you feel you need more help with fuelling your sport and exercise and optimising your performance, I highly recommend that you invest in seeing a Sports Dietitian. This is an area which I believe is often undervalued when it comes to achieving optimal performance and it could just be the key to your own sporting success.

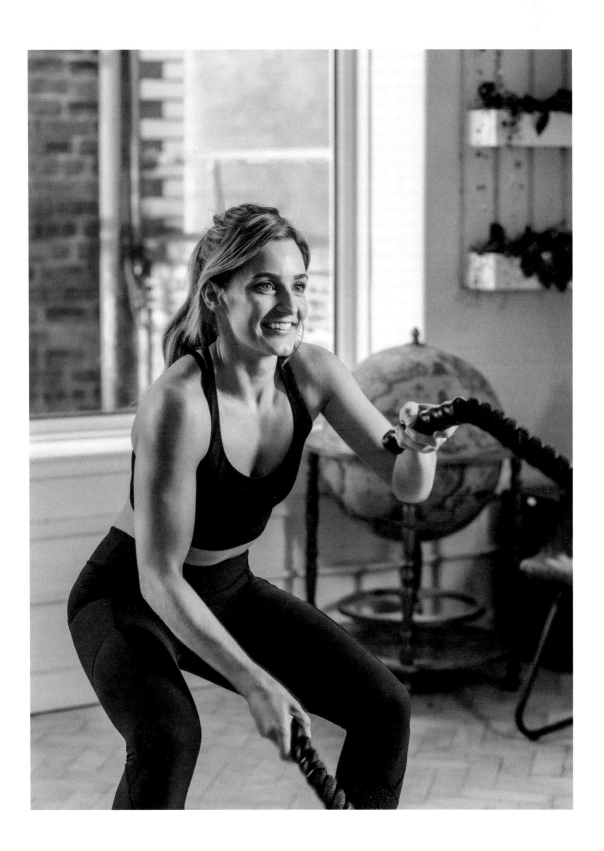

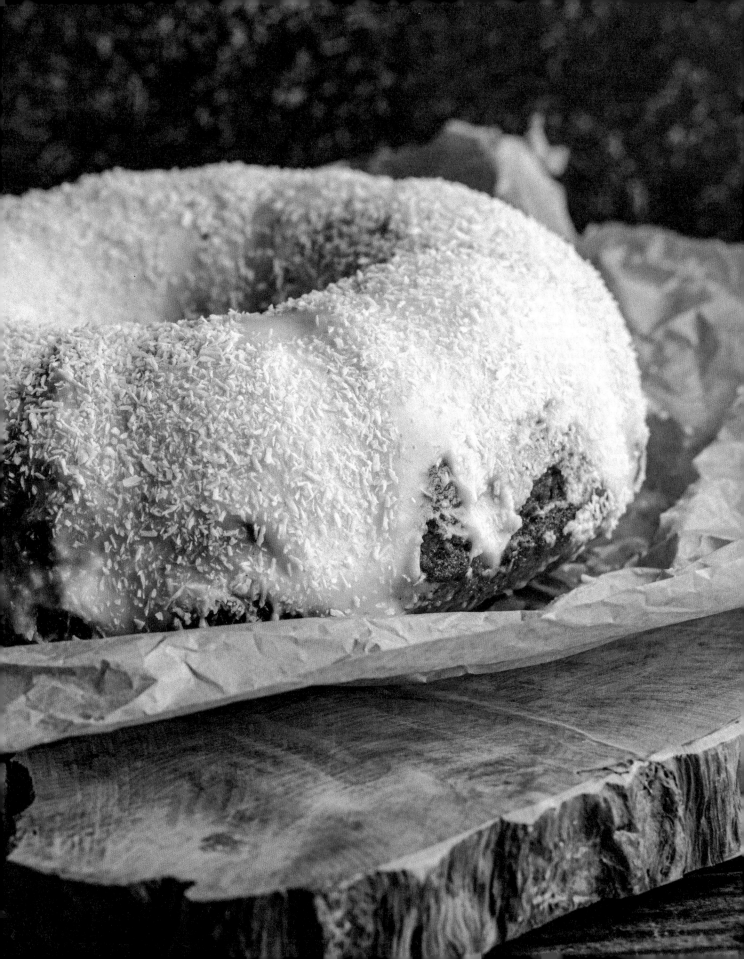

Recipes

Now this is where the fun really begins!

In this section, I am sharing all my favourite recipes to inspire you to get in the kitchen and create some delicious meals and snacks!

Many of the recipes can be easily adapted to be made suitable for vegetarians, vegans, and those with a gluten or lactose intolerance by making some simple ingredient swaps! Just make sure you double check the packaging of a product before you buy to make sure that it specifies that it's 100% gluten-free, lactose-free, vegan or vegetarian.

Useful Kitchen Equipment to Invest In

» Good quality kitchen knives

» Food processor

» Hand blender/Immersion hand mixer

» Different types of airtight containers for taking your food on the go, as well as ones suitable for home freezing

» Ziplock bags

» Kitchen scales

» Measuring cups

» Measuring spoons

I've mentioned a few times that I'm a big fan of batch cooking, so that I have lots of extra portions to pop into the freezer for the days I'm short of time or lack the motivation to cook. Many of the recipes can easily be doubled up to make a larger batch if you like. Although making a larger batch may take that little bit of extra time, I can guarantee that it will save you more time and money in the long-term, and it's a really great way of helping to keep you on track with eating well.

I love a spacious, clutter-free kitchen so I don't have a lot of kitchen gadgets, but there are a couple of essential pieces of equipment that I don't feel I could do without and that will come in handy for you if you are trying out these recipes!

Note: The temperatures indicated in the recipes are all based on using a fan-assisted oven. If you are using a conventional oven, increase the temperature by 20°C. (See the back of the book for a temperature conversion chart.)

Breakfast

Breakfast. My favourite meal of the day. I always look forward to having breakfast and love starting my day with something really delicious. I really believe that making the time to eat a nourishing and delicious breakfast in the morning has the power to set you up for the day ahead. It can boost your energy levels and encourage healthy habits to continue as the day goes on.

I have created a bunch of healthy breakfast recipes for you – both sweet and savoury – to suit your taste buds. There are plenty which are great for those mornings when time is a bit limited, such as delicious overnight oats that you can prepare the night before and take on the go, as well as smoothies that can be made in seconds. There are also several which are suitable for those weekend days when you aren't rushing to get out the door, and you have that little extra time to rustle up something a little bit more extravagant.

COCONUT & BERRY BREAKFAST CRUMBLE

Did someone say dessert for breakfast? If you're anything like me and prefer something sweet for breakfast in the morning, this recipe is the one for you. It's a great alternative way of using oats, it's packed full of fibre, and it can sort you out for breakfast for a few days if you keep it well-sealed in the fridge. I love serving this up with some Greek yoghurt to add in that protein punch, and it's great for keeping me going until lunch and for that post-workout fuel if you're like me and like to exercise in the morning. This is also lovely as a healthy dessert, too. (See page 147.)

LOADED AVOCADO & ZESTY VEGGIE TOAST

This recipe is so tasty and light. It's provides a great source of plant-based protein and fibre and is packed full of satisfying complex carbs and lots of heart-healthy fats. It's a great way to dress up your toast in the morning and provides a delicious and nutritious start to your day. (See page 148.)

SPINACH, FETA & RED PEPPER MUFFINS

These are great for breakkie-on-the-go or for a healthy snack. They contain protein and healthy fats, are a great fibre source and have lots of vitamins and minerals. I love making a big batch and using them for a pre-workout snack before I head to the gym in the morning. (See page 149.)

LEMON & BLUEBERRY PANCAKES

This is one of my favourite breakfast recipes to make at the weekend. Pancakes always remind me of my lovely Gran as I used to make them all the time with her when I was a kid. This recipe is much healthier than the ones we used to make, but I promise they're still delicious. These pancakes are packed full of nutrients and fibre, and if you also serve them up with some Greek yoghurt, you'll get that extra hit of protein to help keep you satisfied until lunch. You can also make these pancakes for a healthy dessert as well. (See page 150.)

POACHED EGGS & AVOCADO SALSA ON TOASTED RYE BREAD

This one is definitely in my top 10. This breakfast dish is so quick and easy to make, and a great recipe to serve up if you have some friends coming round for brunch. Poached eggs are my favourite, but this recipe also goes great with boiled, fried and scrambled eggs, too. (See page 152.)

PEACH & GRANOLA TOAST

Don't knock it before you try it. It's a little bit different, but I love this recipe. It's something I often like to have in the summer – it's so light and refreshing, and the natural sweetness from the peach makes it feel like a real treat. It's a great source of nutrients including complex carbs, fibre, calcium and protein to name but a few, providing a nourishing and delicious breakfast. (See page 153.)

CRANBERRY & APRICOT GRANOLA

I absolutely love granola but finding a ready-made one in the supermarkets that isn't full of added sugar is difficult. Making your own can be easy and it means you are in full control of how much sweetness you add. I've made this recipe with some maple syrup and some dried fruit to keep it sweet. I love having mine served with ice cold milk or sprinkled on top of thick Greek yoghurt. (See page 154.)

SWEET OMELETTE

A sweet twist on a classic savoury favourite. I absolutely love savoury omelettes and find them a great way of packing in a bunch of veggies at breakfast time. I only created this sweet version one day when I had no fresh vegetables left in my fridge but still fancied an omelette for breakfast. The omelette is more like a fluffy soufflé and can be made quickly and easily if you have a hand blender for whisking up the egg whites. If not, you have to have a little patience if you're going to prepare it by hand. I usually serve this one up with some warm berries, Greek yoghurt and lots of cinnamon. (See page 155.)

MANGO, RASPBERRY & COCONUT CHIA PUDDING

This is a delicious and healthy recipe that you can easily prepare the night before, so it's ready to grab and go in the morning. It's packed full of nutrients and is great for those of you following a plant-based diet. The chia seeds are a great source of plant-based protein, containing all the essential amino acids we need and providing you with a source of Omega-3 fats. (See page 156.)

SPICY BAKED BEANS

Who doesn't love baked beans on toast? This meal really reminds me of being a kid, as well as my uni days when I needed a cheap and easy meal option. However, many of the tinned baked beans you can buy in the supermarkets nowadays have a lot of sugar added to them, so I decided to create my own healthy version. This recipe is packed full of flavour and after you've tried it, you'll not want to buy a ready-made tin of baked beans ever again! (See page 157.)

BLACK BEAN BREAKFAST BURRITO

I absolutely love Mexican food, so this Mexican-inspired recipe is easily one of my favourites. This healthy recipe can make a nourishing meal which is suitable for breakfast, lunch or dinner. Not only that, but the bean mixtures can easily be prepared the night before to save you time in the morning, and the wraps can be enjoyed cold, too. These burritos are full of protein and a great source of vitamins, minerals and fibre. (See page 158.)

CREAMY MUSHROOMS ON TOAST

I made my own version of mushrooms on toast unintentionally one day when I fancied something savoury for breakfast but had very little in the way of ingredients in my fridge, so I had to be a little creative. This is now one of my favourite quick and easy breakfast options to make on a regular basis. Did you know that mushrooms naturally contain some Vitamin D but, similar to humans, mushrooms can naturally produce Vitamin D, too, following exposure to sunlight? I always look for mushrooms which are advertised as being a good source of Vitamin D to boost my levels of this important nutrient. (See page 159.)

CHICKPEA & AVOCADO BRUSCHETTA

This recipe can easily be made suitable for vegetarians and vegans by leaving out the cheese, and I absolutely love making it if I have family and friends round for brunch. It's so simple and easy to make, and the quantities can quickly be increased to serve more people. (See page 160.)

POACHED EGGS & QUINOA-STUFFED MUSHROOMS

This breakfast treat is a lighter alternative to the traditional eggs on toast or muffins, yet so unbelievably filling. The quinoa adds an extra protein punch, providing a great plant-based source of all the essential amino acids we need. If you've not mastered the art of poaching an egg yet, this also goes great with boiled or scrambled eggs, too. (See page 162.)

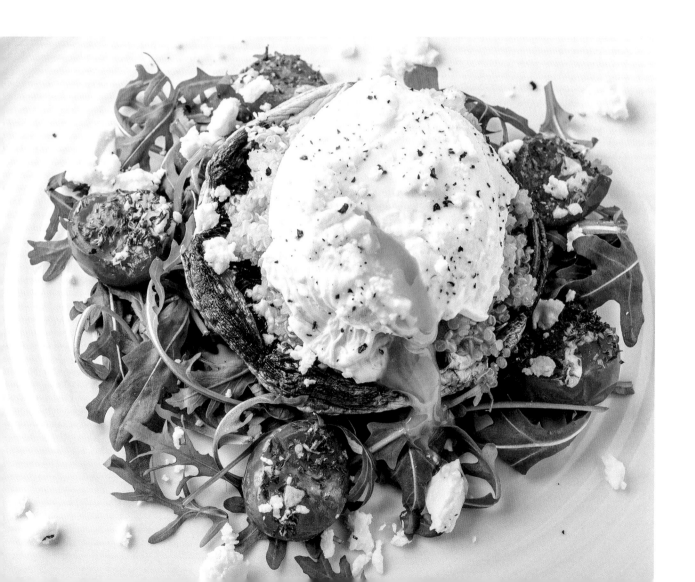

OAT BREAKKIES

Anyone who knows me knows just how much I love my porridge. I eat it most days, have done so for years, and I'm still not tired of it. There are literally so many ways that you can make it, and you can rarely go wrong. Not only that, but porridge is a super quick and simple breakfast to make, too.

Oats are a great source of complex carbohydrates which give you that slow release of energy that can keep you going until lunch. They are also rich in a type of fibre known as beta-glucan, which has been recognised as having blood cholesterol-lowering properties! What's not to love?

BANANA & CINNAMON OATS

What I love about this recipe is that the mashed banana gives all the sweetness the oats need without having to add any honey or syrup. It's packed full of nutrients, and the chia seeds add a great source of plant-based protein and Omega-3 fats. If you want a little extra protein, you can always stir in some nut butter too. (See page 164.)

BANANA & BLUEBERRY OATS

I think that just the amazing colour of this bowl of oats already tells you that it's going to taste delicious. I like adding the blueberries during cooking because I think their flavour is released even more, making for a really tasty breakfast. This is another recipe where I feel the oats really are sweet enough, thanks to the natural sweetness of the fruit, that nothing else is needed to sweeten them up. I love to add a sprinkle of pistachios to the top for that extra bit of crunchiness! (See page 165.)

POMEGRANATE & PUMPKIN SEED OATS

This is also a definite favourite of mine – but I could probably say that about all porridge recipes! The flavours in this go great together, and the pomegranate adds a delicious crunch! I love adding flaxseeds to my food whenever I can, too – I often add it to porridge, yoghurt, smoothies, over salads and even to stews and sauces! They're a powerhouse of nutrition providing a great source of fibre to support good digestive habits and are also a source of Omega-3 fats! (See page 166.)

PEANUT BUTTER & CHIA SEED JAM OATS

Come on, who doesn't love the traditional favourite combo of PB&J? Although this combination is normally served up on a sandwich or toast, it goes just as well (if not better!) with or added to a bowl of porridge. (See page 167.)

APPLE & CINNAMON OATS

Now if I didn't call this recipe my absolute favourite, then people would definitely have something to say about it! This is the recipe I have been making for years and have shared how to make it lots of times on my social media channels. So many people have now told me that they've tried making it themselves and have also found a new favourite. It's like Christmas in a bowl. But who says you can't eat it all year round? I certainly do! (See page 168.)

BERRY BURSTING OATS

The clue is in the name. The colour from all the berries in this recipe gives the oats an absolutely amazing colour and with that, a truly delicious flavour. (See page 169.)

LEMON & BLUEBERRY OVERNIGHT OATS

Overnight oats are such a great idea if you are someone who is always in a rush in the morning. You can prepare them the night before, pop them in a container and grab and go the next morning – just don't forget a spoon! This recipe has a zesty, refreshing flavour, and is packed with protein thanks to the Greek yoghurt and chia seeds. (See page 170.)

TROPICAL PARADISE OVERNIGHT OATS

This is another take on overnight oats. This one tastes like summer and the flavour combination reminds me of a fruity cocktail. Sadly it won't take you to a real tropical paradise, but you can at least close your eyes and pretend you're there, right? (See page 171.)

CARROT CAKE OVERNIGHT OATS

Who wouldn't like cake for breakfast? This delicious number tastes just like the real deal (well, almost!), and it's packed full of nourishing ingredients. Not only that, but you're also getting one of your five-a-day veggies in there, too. This recipe is so filling and will help keep you going all the way to lunch. (See page 172.)

BANANA & WALNUT OVERNIGHT OATS

Another favourite of mine if I need a breakfast on-the-go. You can always play around with the ingredients in this one, too, and try adding different nuts or seeds to suit your taste buds. I also like adding some cacao powder through this to give a rich, chocolatey taste. (See page 173.)

SMOOTHIES

Smoothies are a really great way to pack in a bunch of nutrients and if you're someone who doesn't have much time in the morning, a smoothie can be your solution. Not only that, but they can be a great option if you're someone who doesn't have a great appetite for food in the morning, helping you to get some nutrition in liquid form.

I've provided some delicious smoothie recipes for you to try, but if you are keen to be creative and want to try and make your own, then it's really important for you to pack it with food sources from each of the five different food groups if you can. (See page 174.)

Don't be afraid to be creative! You can rarely go wrong when it comes to making smoothies, so give it a go by following the same idea of how you should be "Building a Balanced Plate".

1. FLUID: Your base ingredient could be water, milk, coconut milk, almond milk, soya milk, coconut water, etc. Choosing a dairy or fortified dairy-free alternative option can provide you with a good source of calcium and many other nutrients.

2. COMPLEX CARBS: The only appropriate option here tends to be oats. I like to include oats often when I'm making smoothies to help provide that slow release of energy.

3. PROTEIN: This could be milk, Greek yoghurt, Quark, Whey Protein, etc. Protein should be included at each meal to promote the growth and repair of body tissues.

4. FRUITS and VEGETABLES: This is where you can really be creative. Add your choice of fruit and vegetables and aim for a few different kinds in each smoothie to get lots of different vitamins and minerals. Generally speaking, the more colour, the more nutrients! I usually like to use frozen fruit and vegetables for smoothies. They tend to keep the smoothie nice and cold, which saves adding any ice to it, and they can also give the smoothie a lovely creamy texture. Not only that, but frozen fruit can be a little bit cheaper, too. I'd much prefer to keep the lovely fresh versions for eating and choose frozen fruit for smoothies, since they're just going to be mixed up in a blender anyway.

5. HEALTHY FATS: Remember, healthy fats are good for keeping us feeling full and provide a number of health benefits. Try adding some avocado to your smoothie or even a spoonful of nut butter, or a small handful of nuts and seeds.

Coconut & Berry Breakfast Crumble

Serves: 3-4 | **Difficulty:** Easy | **Prep time:** 10 min. | **Cook time:** 25-30 min. | Suitable for vegetarians

1. Preheat oven to 180°C (fan).

2. Place all berry ingredients into a saucepan and heat at low-medium heat for approx. 3 minutes. The berries should be soft and covered evenly with honey, vanilla essence and the spices. Set aside in the saucepan.

3. To make the crumble topping, in a bowl, mix together the oats, flour, dried coconut and hazelnuts.

4. Add in the coconut oil and the 2 tbsp honey and mix together until well combined.

5. Spread the berry mixture evenly along the bottom of 8x4in. baking pan or ramekin. If using an alternative pan, just make sure it is at least 3/4 full with the berry mixture.

6. Top the berries evenly with the crumble mixture.

7. Crush the toasted, flaked almonds in your hands and sprinkle them evenly on top of the crumble topping.

8. Sprinkle extra desiccated coconut as desired over the top of the crumble.

9. Place the baking pan in the oven and bake for 25-30 minutes, until the crumble looks golden on top.

10. Serve it up with some Greek yoghurt on the side.

Ingredients

» *Berry Filling*

6 handfuls of fresh mixed berries

2 tbsp honey

2 tsp vanilla essence

1 tsp cinnamon

1 tsp nutmeg

» *Coconut Crumble Topping*

150g oats

1 tbsp plain flour

2-3 tbsp dried coconut

2 tbsp chopped roasted hazelnuts

3 tsp melted coconut oil

2 tbsp honey

1 tbsp toasted flaked almonds

Extra desiccated coconut for sprinkle over top

» *To Serve*

1-2 tbsp Greek yoghurt

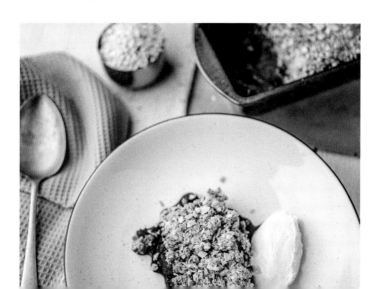

Loaded Avocado and Zesty Veggie Toast

Serves: 1 | **Difficulty:** Easy | **Prep time:** 5 min. | **Cook time:** 10 min. | Suitable for vegetarians

Ingredients

2 slices sourdough bread

1 garlic clove, halved lengthways

Zest of 1/2 lemon

Juice of 1/2 lemon

1/2 avocado, mashed

Salt and pepper, to taste

20g frozen broad beans

30g frozen peas

2 cherry tomatoes, halved

1/2 tsp chilli flakes

1/2 tbsp Extra Virgin Olive Oil

10g crumbled feta (optional)

1. Rub one side of the slices of bread with the garlic.

2. In a bowl, mix together the lemon juice and avocado and season with salt and pepper.

3. Cook the broad beans and peas as per the package instructions.

4. Meanwhile, toast the bread.

5. Top the garlic side of the toast with the avocado mix, followed by the peas and broad beans and the cherry tomatoes.

6. Sprinkle with the chilli flakes and crumbled feta, drizzle the extra virgin olive oil over the toast, sprinkling the lemon zest as a final touch.

7. Add extra seasoning if desired.

Spinach, Feta & Red Pepper Muffins

Serves: 12 | **Difficulty:** Easy | **Prep time:** 10 min. | **Cook time:** 20 min. | Suitable for vegetarians

1. Preheat oven to 200°C.

2. Line a muffin tray with paper muffin cups.

3. In a frying pan, heat 1 tbsp olive oil over low-medium heat.

4. Sauté the onion and pepper until softened.

5. Add the seeds to the pan and sauté for a further 1-2 minutes, stirring regularly. Remove from the heat and set aside.

6. In a bowl, combine the egg, milk and the remaining 3 tbsp oil using a fork.

7. In a separate bowl, sift in the flour. Add the mixed herbs, sea salt and black pepper, spinach and feta cheese and mix together.

8. Add the onion and pepper to this bowl and mix thoroughly.

9. Add the wet ingredients to the dry ingredients and combine well.

10. Spoon the mixture evenly into the 12 muffin cups.

11. Sprinkle the top of each one with the extra seeds.

12. Bake for approx. 25-30 minutes or until golden brown on top and a knife or cake tester comes out clean.

13. Top each muffin with approx. 1 tsp butter while they're still hot and sprinkle some parmesan over the tops.

14. Transfer the muffins onto a wire rack to cool.

15. They can be enjoyed either warm or cold!

Ingredients

4 tbsp olive oil

1/2 onion, finely chopped

1 red pepper, finely chopped

1/2 tbsp pumpkin seeds (plus some extra to top)

1/2 tbsp sunflower seeds (plus some extra to top)

1 egg

200ml milk

300g wholemeal self-rising flour

2 tsp mixed herbs

Salt and pepper to season

Large handful of spinach, finely chopped

50g crumbled feta cheese

1 tbsp parmesan to finish

Butter to finish (optional)

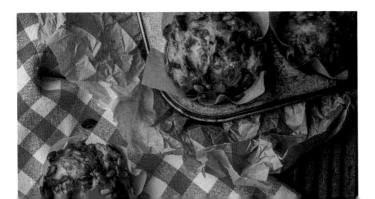

Lemon & Blueberry Pancakes

Serves: 2 | **Difficulty:** Easy | **Prep time:** 15 min. | **Cook time:** 10 min. | Suitable for vegetarians

Ingredients

100g plain wholemeal flour

2 tsp baking powder

Pinch of salt

1 egg

150ml milk

Zest of 1/2 lemon

Juice of 1/2 lemon

60g blueberries

1/2 tbsp butter

Honey/maple syrup to serve (approx. 1 tbsp)

Optional: Greek yoghurt to serve

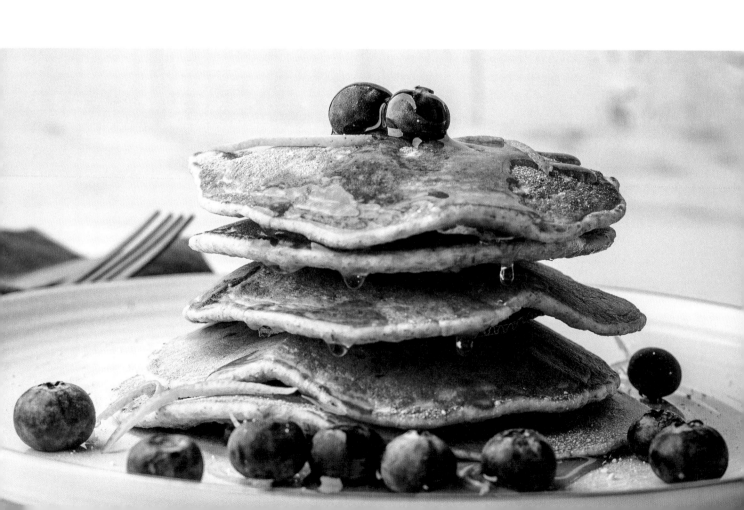

1. In a large bowl, mix together flour, baking powder and a pinch of salt.

2. In a cup, beat the egg and milk.

3. Create a well in the middle of the flour mixture.

4. Add in the egg and milk mixture to the well in the flour mixture and beat together until a smooth batter is formed.

5. Add the lemon juice and lemon zest and stir together.

6. Gently stir in half of the blueberries, to make sure the blueberries don't burst.

7. Leave to stand for 10 minutes to get rid of any air bubbles.

8. Heat the butter in a large non-stick frying pan.

9. Drop in 1 heaping tbsp of the batter mixture onto the pan. Add in about 2-3 tbsp if you can to cook a few at the same time. Just make sure not to overcrowd the pan as it will make it difficult to flip the pancakes.

10. Cook on one side until the underside has browned and bubbles have started to form on the top surface. Flip the pancakes to allow them to cook on the other side. The pancakes are ready when they have developed a light crust.

11. Remove from the pan and continue, following the same process until all the batter is used up.

12. Make a stack of pancakes and top with the remaining blueberries.

13. Drizzle over some honey or maple syrup and a dusting of icing sugar and serve with a dollop of Greek yoghurt for that extra protein boost!

Poached Eggs & Avocado Salsa on Toasted Rye

Serves: 1 | **Difficulty:** Easy | **Prep time:** 5 min. | **Cook time:** 5-10 min.

Ingredients

Prepare the Avocado Salsa (See recipe in Dips & Spreads.)

1/2 tbsp vinegar

2 slices rye bread

2 free-range eggs

Sea salt and black pepper to season

Optional: Sprinkle of Dukkah (Egyptian Spice)

1. Bring a large pot of water to boiling and add the vinegar.

2. Turn the heat down to a slight simmer.

3. Crack the eggs into two separate cups.

4. Stir the water with a slotted spoon, forming a gentle whirlpool – this helps keep the eggs together.

5. Gently pour the eggs into the centre of the whirlpool one at a time, making sure that the heat is low enough so that only a few bubbles are rising.

6. Allow the eggs to cook for approx. 3-4 minutes or until the egg white has set.

7. In the meantime, while the eggs are cooking, toast the rye bread, then top one side of it with a layer of the avocado salsa.

8. Take the poached eggs out of the water using a slotted spoon and place one on top of each piece of toast and avocado salsa,

9. Season as desired and top with a sprinkle of Dukkah.

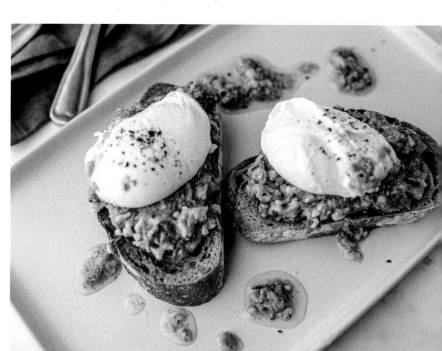

Peach & Granola Toast

Serves: 1 | **Difficulty:** Easy | **Total time:** 5 min.

....

Ingredients

2 slices wholegrain bread

100g low-fat plain yoghurt

1 tsp honey (optional)

6-8 peach slices

1-2 tsp granola

1 tsp chia seeds

1. Toast the bread as desired.

2. Meanwhile, in a bowl, mix together the plain yoghurt with the honey then spread it over one side of the toast.

3. Top the bread with the peach slices and a sprinkle of granola and chia seeds.

Cranberry & Apricot Granola

Serves: 5-6 | **Difficulty:** Easy | **Prep time:** 5 min. | **Cook time:** 30 min. | Suitable for vegetarians and vegans

Ingredients

150g rolled oats

1 tbsp coconut oil

2 tbsp maple syrup

1 tsp vanilla essence

25g sunflower seeds

2 tbsp sesame seeds

25g pumpkin seeds

20g flaxseeds

1 tsp cinnamon

1 tbsp toasted flaked almonds

25g coconut flakes

25g dried cranberries

25g chopped dried apricots

1. Preheat oven to 150°C.

2. In a large bowl, mix together the oats, coconut oil, maple syrup and vanilla essence in a large bowl.

3. Add the sunflower seeds, sesame seeds, pumpkin seeds, golden linseeds, cinnamon, toasted flaked almonds and mix well.

4. Cover a baking tray with baking parchment.

5. Tip the granola mixture onto the baking sheet and spread evenly.

6. Put the baking tray in the oven and bake for 10 minutes.

7. Remove the baking tray from the oven and sprinkle on the coconut flakes and dried fruit. Shake the tray so the mixture loosens from the baking parchment and the coconut and dried fruit gets mixed thoroughly. Bake for another 5-10 minutes until the granola has browned all over. Be sure to keep an eye on it as not all ovens bake at the same speed!

8. Remove the granola from the baking tray and scrape onto a flat tray to cool. Store in an airtight container.

Sweet Omelette

Serves: 2 | **Difficulty:** Easy | **Prep time:** 10 min. | **Cook time:** 10 min.

1. Heat the oven grill/broiler to high heat.

2. Separate the egg whites from the yolks and put them into two separate bowls.

3. Beat the egg yolks together.

4. Add the yoghurt and vanilla extract to the yolks and mix thoroughly.

5. Beat the egg whites to form soft peaks using a hand mixer if you have one.

6. Add the yolk and yoghurt mixture to the egg whites. Fold them together gradually and gently until well combined.

7. Add the butter to a medium-sized frying pan and heat at medium-high heat.

8. Pour the omelette mixture into the frying pan, ensuring that it's spread evenly.

9. Cook the mixture until it's golden brown on the bottom. Remove from the heat.

10. Place the frying pan under the oven grill for a few minutes (be sure to keep the handle away from the grill!) and cook until the omelette is set and golden.

11. Turn the omelette out onto a plate and add your chosen fruit.

12. Serve with a side of Greek yoghurt, top with the granola, a drizzle of honey or maple syrup if desired, and a dusting of cinnamon.

Ingredients

» *For the Omelette*

2 medium eggs

2 tbsp low-fat Greek yoghurt

1 tsp vanilla extract

1 tsp butter

» *For the Topping*

2-4 tbsp yoghurt (I use low-fat Greek yoghurt)

Handful of mixed berries or 1/2 banana

1-2 tsp honey or maple syrup

1 tbsp granola

1/2 tsp cinnamon

Mango, Raspberry & Coconut Chia Pudding

Serves: 2 | **Difficulty:** Easy | **Prep time:** 10 min. | Suitable for vegetarians

Ingredients

200ml unsweetened coconut milk

1 tsp vanilla essence

1 tbsp chia seeds

3 tsp honey

80g mango

80g raspberries

Desiccated coconut to serve

1. In a bowl, mix together the coconut milk, vanilla essence, chia seeds and 2 tsp honey.

2. Refrigerate overnight if possible, or until the mixture has formed a thick consistency.

3. In a food processor or blender, add the mango and pulse until smooth.

4. In a bowl, combine the raspberries with the remaining 1 tsp of honey. Crush the raspberries slightly with a fork.

5. In a suitable jar or container, layer up the ingredients starting with the chia seed pudding mix first, followed by the raspberry puree, then the mango puree.

6. Top with a sprinkle of desiccated coconut to serve.

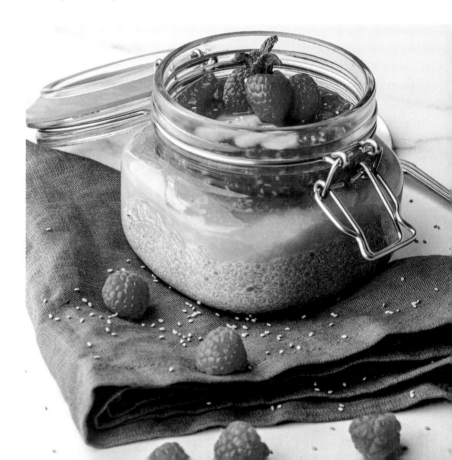

Spicy Baked Beans

Serves: 1 | **Difficulty:** Easy | **Prep time:** 10 min. | **Cook time:** 10 min. | Suitable for vegetarians and vegans

1. In a medium frying pan, heat the oil on medium heat.

2. Add the onion, garlic and dried coriander to the pan and cook for a few minutes until the onion is soft, stirring constantly so the garlic doesn't burn.

3. Add the haricot beans, tomato passata/strained tomatoes, chilli (or chilli flakes), Worcestershire sauce and maple syrup and mix together.

4. Season as desired with salt and pepper and cook for a further 3-5 minutes at medium heat, stirring regularly.

5. Meanwhile, toast the bread.

6. Top the toast with the bean mixture and grated cheese.

Ingredients

2 tsp olive oil

1/4 red onion, finely chopped

1 garlic clove, crushed

1/2 tsp dried coriander

150g haricot beans, drained and rinsed

100ml tomato passata/strained tomatoes

1/2 fresh red chilli, finely chopped (or 1/2 tsp chilli flakes)

1 tsp Worcestershire sauce or soy sauce (choose vegetarian/vegan varieties if desired)

1 tsp maple syrup

Salt and pepper, to season

2 slices wholegrain toast

20g cheddar cheese, grated (optional)

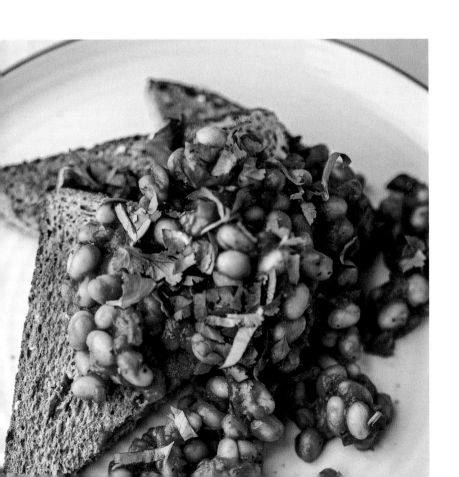

Black Bean Breakfast Burrito

Serves: 2 | **Difficulty:** Easy | **Prep time:** 10 min. | **Cook time:** 5 min.

Ingredients

200g black beans, drained and rinsed

1/2 red onion, finely chopped

1 garlic clove, crushed

Juice of 1/2 lime

1/2 red pepper, diced

1/2 tsp chilli flakes or 1/2 fresh chilli, finely diced

Small handful of fresh coriander, finely chopped

4 cherry tomatoes, finely chopped

Salt and black pepper, to season

4 medium eggs

2 small wholemeal tortilla wraps

1/2 tbsp butter

1/2 avocado, diced

20g low fat cheddar cheese, grated

Optional: 2 tbsp of beans from my Spicy Baked Beans recipe

1. In a small bowl, mix together the black beans, red onion, garlic, lime juice, red pepper, chilli flakes (or fresh chilli), coriander and tomatoes, Season with salt and pepper to taste and set aside.

2. Crack the eggs into a bowl and whisk together with a fork. Add in half the cheese and season as required with salt and pepper.

3. Heat a medium frying pan to medium heat and add the butter.

4. Add the egg mixture to the pan and stir continuously with a wooden spoon, lifting and folding from the bottom of the pan, making sure the mixture doesn't burn.

5. Remove the pan from the heat. The texture should be nice and velvety.

6. To assemble a burrito, add a line of scrambled egg down the middle of each tortilla wrap. Top with the black bean mixture and 2 tbsp of my Spicy Baked Beans if desired. Add some chopped avocado, sprinkle with the remainder of the grated cheese and roll up the tortilla!

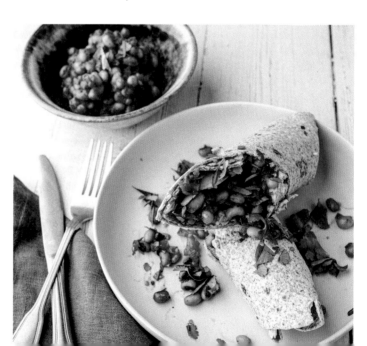

Creamy Mushrooms on Toast

Serves: 1 | **Difficulty:** Easy | **Prep time:** 5 min. | **Cook time:** 5 min.

1. In a medium frying pan, heat the oil over medium heat.

2. Add the onions and garlic to the pan and cook until the onions look transparent. Stir constantly so the garlic doesn't burn.

3. Add the mushrooms to the pan and cook until soft.

4. Stir in the low-fat soft cheese, salt and pepper and tarragon and cook for another 3 minutes, stirring often.

5. Meanwhile, toast the bread.

6. Serve the mushrooms on top of the toast with an extra sprinkle of herbs if desired.

Ingredients

1 tbsp olive oil

1/4 onion, finely diced

1 clove garlic, crushed

80g mushrooms, finely sliced

2 tbsp low-fat soft cheese

Salt and pepper to season

1 tsp tarragon

2 slices wholemeal toast

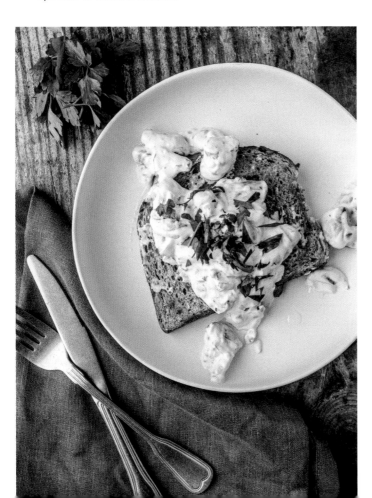

Chickpea & Avocado Bruschetta

Serves: 1 | **Difficulty:** Easy | **Prep time:** 5 min. | **Cook time:** 15 min. | Suitable for vegetarians and vegans

Ingredients

2 slices sourdough bread

5 cherry tomatoes, halved

1-2 tbsp Extra Virgin Olive Oil

Salt and pepper, to taste

1/2 tsp dried oregano

1 garlic clove, crushed

1/4 red onion, finely sliced

Juice of 1/2 lime

3 tbsp chickpeas, drained and rinsed

5 fresh basil leaves, sliced

1/2 avocado, diced

Optional: Crumbled feta or a few slices of mozzarella

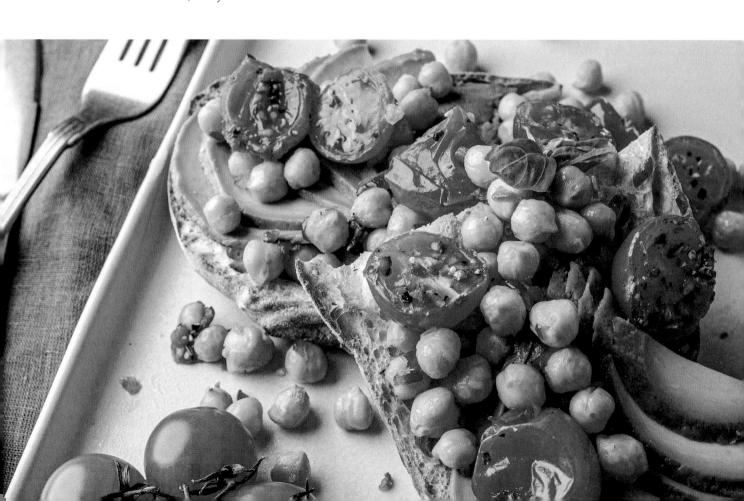

1. Preheat oven to 180°C (fan).

2. Drizzle bread with a small amount of olive oil. (Optional: Cut a clove of garlic lengthways and rub on bread for extra flavour!)

3. Line a baking tray with baking parchment. Add cherry tomatoes and a drizzle of oil, season with salt and pepper and a sprinkle of dried oregano. Place in the oven and heat for a few minutes until the tomatoes soften. Take out and set aside.

4. Line another baking tray with baking parchment. Add the bread and bake it in the oven for 5-10 minutes until golden brown or simply toast in the microwave.

5. Meanwhile, heat 1 tbsp olive oil in a frying pan at medium heat. Add the crushed garlic and red onion to the pan and sauté for approximately 1 minute.

6. Add the lime juice, chickpeas and extra salt and pepper as desired, and sauté for a few more minutes until the ingredients are warmed through.

7. Remove from the heat and stir in the fresh basil.

8. Once the bread is ready, top it with the avocado, the chickpea mixture and the tomatoes.

9. I love topping this dish off with some crumbled feta or mozzarella for some extra flavour!

Poached Eggs & Quinoa-Stuffed Mushrooms

Serves: 1 | **Difficulty:** Easy | **Prep time:** 5 min. | **Cook time:** 25 min.

Ingredients

30g quinoa

100ml vegetable stock

4 cherry tomatoes, halved

1/2-1 tbsp olive oil

1/2 tsp dried parsley

1 large flat mushroom, stalk removed

Handful of rocket leaves

1/2 red onion, finely chopped

1 medium egg

Crumbled feta, to taste

Salt and pepper, to season

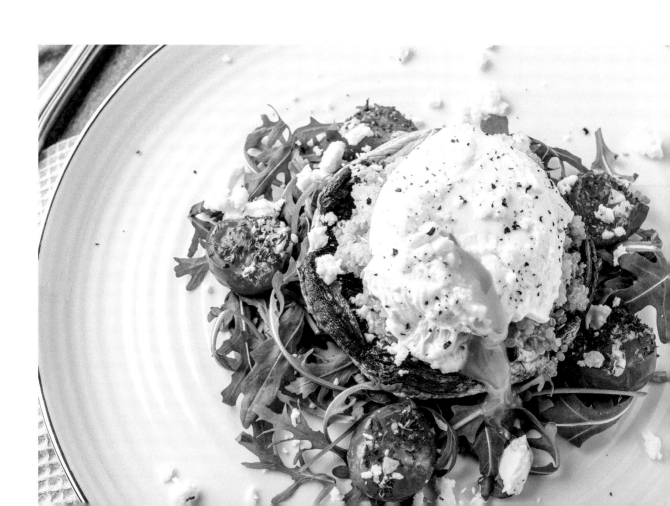

1. Preheat oven to 180°C.

2. Cook the quinoa as per package instructions using vegetable stock.

3. Meanwhile, place the tomatoes and mushroom on a baking tray and drizzle them both with olive oil. Sprinkle some dried parsley over the tomatoes.

4. Bake the mushroom and tomatoes in the oven for approx.. 15 minutes.

5. Add a bed of rocket to your plate and sprinkle red onion over it.

6. After 15 minutes, remove the baking tray from the oven and stuff the mushroom with the quinoa. Return the tray to the oven for another 5 minutes.

7. Meanwhile, to poach the egg – bring a large pot of water to boiling and add the vinegar.

8. Turn the heat down to a slight simmer.

9. Crack the egg into a cup.

10. Stir the water with a slotted spoon, forming a gentle whirlpool – this helps keep the egg together.

11. Gently pour the egg into the centre of the whirlpool, making sure that the heat is low enough so that only a few bubbles are rising.

12. Allow the egg to cook for approx. 3-4 minutes or until the egg white has set.

13. Scatter the tomatoes over the bed of rocket and top it with the mushroom. Once the poached egg is ready, place it on top of the mushroom.

14. Season with extra salt and pepper, if desired and sprinkle over some crumbled feta as a final touch.

OAT BREAKKIES

Banana & Cinnamon Oats

Serves: 1 | **Difficulty:** Easy | **Total time:** 10 min. | Suitable for vegetarians

Ingredients

1 banana, peeled and sliced

40g oats

125mls milk (any kind)

15g chia seeds

1/2 tsp cinnamon

10g toasted, flaked almonds

Sprinkle of desiccated coconut

15g nut butter (optional)

1. Mash half the sliced banana with a fork. Set the other half aside.

2. Add the oats, milk, mashed banana, chia seeds and cinnamon to a small saucepan and stir thoroughly until well combined.

3. Cook over medium heat for 3-5 minutes until the porridge is creamy and has thickened.

4. Spoon the porridge into a bowl and top with the remaining banana slices, a sprinkle of toasted, flaked almonds and desiccated coconut. Top with nut butter, if desired.

Banana & Blueberry Oats

Serves: 1 | **Difficulty:** Easy | **Total time:** 10 min. | Suitable for vegetarians and vegans

1. Mash half the sliced banana with a fork. Set the other half aside.

2. Put the blueberries in a saucepan with a splash of water and cook at medium heat. Heat thoroughly for a couple of minutes until the blueberries become soft and begin to burst.

3. To the same saucepan, add the oats, milk and vanilla essence and stir thoroughly until combined.

4. Cook the oats over medium heat for 3-5 minutes until the porridge is creamy and has thickened. As the oats are cooking, continue to stir often, bursting the blueberries as they become soft. This gives a splash of colour, giving the porridge a lovely purple tone.

5. Spoon the porridge into a bowl and top with the remaining banana and a sprinkle of pistachios.

Ingredients

1 banana, peeled and sliced

40g oats

125ml milk (any kind)

1 tsp vanilla essence

40g blueberries

10g pistachios, finely chopped

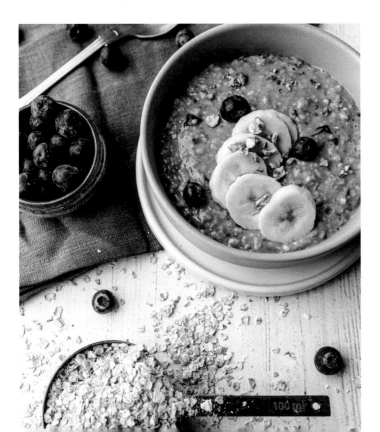

Pomegranate & Pumpkin Seed Oats

Serves: 1 | **Difficulty:** Easy | **Total time:** 10 min. | Suitable for vegetarians

Ingredients

40g oats

125ml milk (almond milk is lovely with this recipe!)

15g chia seeds

1 tsp cinnamon

2 tsp golden linseeds

1 tsp honey

2 tsp pumpkin seeds

20g pomegranate

1. In a small saucepan, add the oats, milk, chia seeds, cinnamon, golden linseeds and honey.

2. Cook the oat mixture over medium heat for 3-5 minutes until the porridge is creamy and has thickened.

3. Spoon the oats into a bowl and top with the pomegranate and a sprinkle of pumpkin seeds.

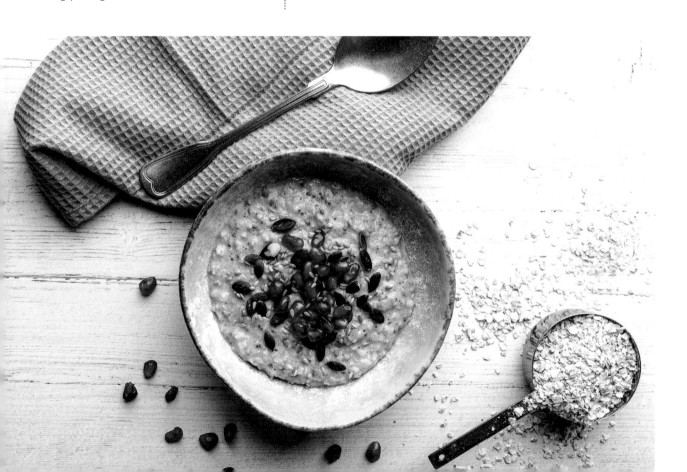

Peanut Butter & Chia Seed Jam Oats

Serves: 1 | **Difficulty:** Easy | **Total time:** 10 min. | Suitable for vegetarians and vegans

1. In a small saucepan, add the banana, oats and milk.

2. Cook the oat mixture over medium heat for 3-5 minutes until the porridge is creamy and has thickened.

3. Spoon the oats into a bowl and stir in the chia jam and the peanut butter.

Ingredients

1/2 banana, mashed

40g oats

125ml milk (any kind)

1/2 tbsp homemade chia seed jam (See my Dips and Spreads section)

1/2 tbsp 100% natural peanut butter

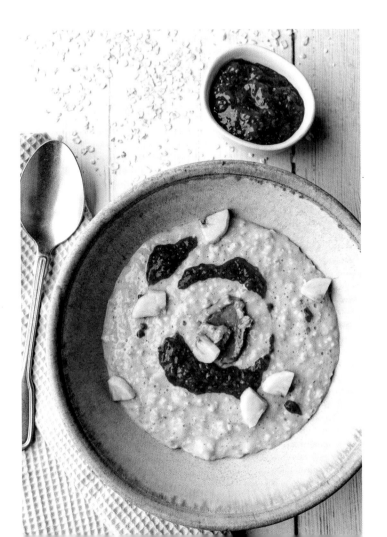

Apple & Cinnamon Oats

Serves: 1 | **Difficulty:** Easy | **Total time:** 10 min. | Suitable for vegetarians

....

Ingredients

1 medium red apple, (1/2 grated and 1/2 chopped into small cubes)

1 tsp cinnamon

1/4 tsp ground nutmeg

40g oats

125ml milk (any kind)

1 tsp maple syrup

1 tsp vanilla essence

10g walnuts (optional)

1. Put the chopped apple with a splash of water in a medium frying pan. Cover the apple with a dusting of cinnamon and nutmeg.

2. In a small saucepan, add the oats, grated apple, milk, maple syrup and vanilla essence.

3. Cook the oat mixture over medium heat for 3-5 minutes until the porridge is creamy and has thickened.

4. At the same time, put the frying pan with the chopped apple on low-medium heat and cook for a few minutes until the chopped apple has softened.

5. Spoon the oat mixture into a bowl and top with the chopped apple and a sprinkle of walnuts, if preferred.

6. Top with a little more cinnamon or maple syrup if desired.

Berry Bursting Oats

Serves: 1 | **Difficulty:** Easy | **Total time:** 10 min. | Suitable for vegetarians

1. Place all the berries in a bowl and mash them with a fork until pulped. This can be done quicker in a food processor.

2. In a small saucepan, add the oats, milk, berry pulp, chia seeds and honey.

3. Cook the oat mixture over medium heat for 3-5 minutes until the porridge is creamy and has thickened.

4. 4. Spoon the oats into a bowl and top with extra berries and chia seeds, if desired, and add a sprinkle of chopped hazelnuts and pumpkin seeds for a final touch.

Ingredients

20g strawberries – tops removed and quartered

20g raspberries

20g blueberries

40g oats

125ml milk (any kind)

1 tbsp chia seeds (extra for topping)

1 tsp honey

Extra berries for topping (optional)

15g chopped hazelnuts

Sprinkle of pumpkin seeds

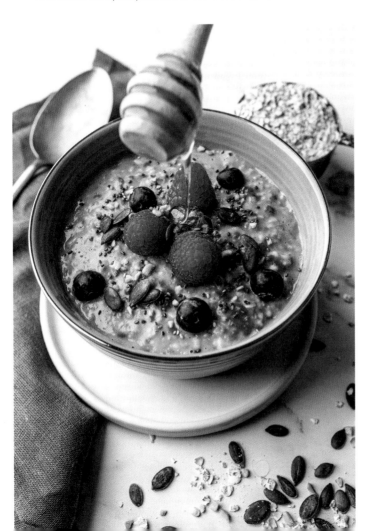

Lemon & Blueberry Overnight Oats

Serves: 1 | **Difficulty:** Easy | **Total time:** 10 min. | Suitable for vegetarians

....

Ingredients

50g Greek yoghurt

125ml coconut milk

1 tsp honey

1/2 tsp vanilla essence

1/2 tsp lemon juice + 1/2 tsp lemon zest

40g oats

10g chia seeds

1 tsp desiccated coconut plus more for topping, if desired

40g blueberries

1. In a bowl, combine the yoghurt, milk, honey, vanilla essence and lemon juice. Taste the mixture and add more lemon juice, if desired.

2. To the same bowl, add the oats, chia seeds and a sprinkle of dried coconut and mix together until well blended.

3. Spoon approximately 1/4 of the mixture into a jar or airtight container before adding a layer of blueberries. Repeat this process until all the oat mixture and blueberries are finished.

4. Store in the fridge overnight.

5. Serve with a sprinkle of lemon zest and desiccated coconut.

Tropical Paradise Overnight Oats

Serves: 1 | **Difficulty:** Easy | **Total time:** 10 min. | Suitable for vegetarians

1. Combine all but the last two ingredients in a bowl.
2. Put the mixture into a jar or airtight container and refrigerate overnight.
3. Top with coconut flakes in the morning and enjoy.

Ingredients

40g oats

50-100mls milk (any kind)

1/2 tbsp chia seeds

1 tsp maple syrup

1 tbsp Greek yoghurt

1/2 tsp vanilla extract

1/2 banana, mashed

1 passion fruit

20g pineapple, finely chopped

20g mango, finely chopped

1/2 tbsp coconut flakes

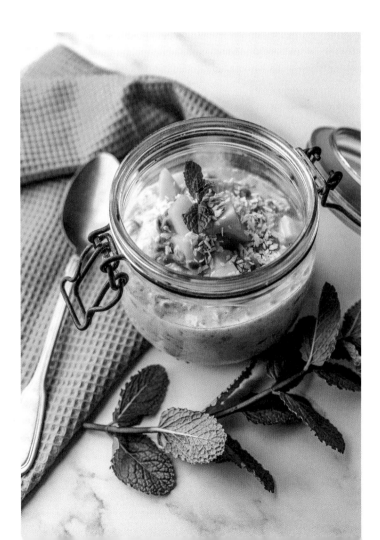

Carrot Cake Overnight Oats

Serves: 1 | **Difficulty:** Easy | **Total time:** 15 min.

Ingredients

100ml milk (almond milk is lovely for this recipe!)

40g oats

1 small carrot, grated

50g Greek yoghurt

1 tsp vanilla essence

1 1/2 tbsp maple syrup

1 tsp cinnamon

1/2 tsp nutmeg

15g raisins

1/2 tbsp low-fat cream cheese

1 tbsp chia seeds

40g chopped walnuts

1. Combine all the ingredients in a large bowl.

2. Pour into an airtight container and refrigerate overnight.

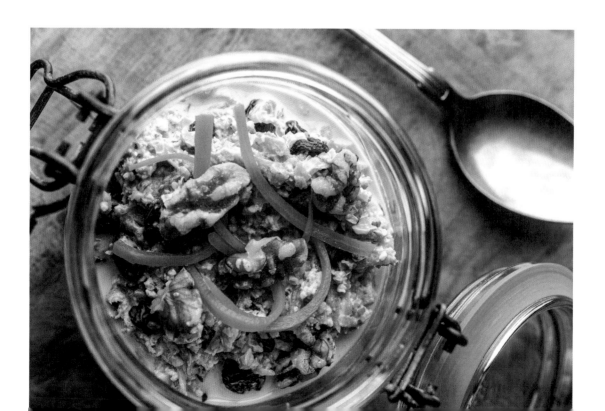

Banana & Walnut Overnight Oats

Serves: 1 | **Difficulty:** Easy | **Total time:** 10 min. | Suitable for vegetarians and vegans

Ingredients

1 banana, mashed

40g oats

100ml milk (any kind)

1/2 tsp vanilla essence

1/2 tsp cinnamon

1 tsp maple syrup or honey

20g raisins

1 tsp ground flaxseeds

15g pumpkin seeds

10g walnuts

1/2 tbsp cacao powder (optional)

1. In a large bowl, add all the ingredients and mix well.
2. Put the mixture into a jar or airtight container and keep in the refrigerator overnight.

SMOOTHIES

Berry Boom Smoothie

Serves: 1 | **Difficulty:** Easy | **Total time:** 5 min. | Suitable for vegetarians

Ingredients

200ml milk (any kind)

1 handful spinach leaves

1 ripe banana, sliced (and frozen, if possible)

40g frozen raspberries

40g frozen blueberries

40g frozen strawberries

1 tsp honey (or maple syrup)

1 tsp vanilla essence

1 tbsp low-fat Greek yoghurt

1/2 tbsp chia seeds

Handful of ice (if desired)

1. Add all ingredients in a blender and blend until smooth.

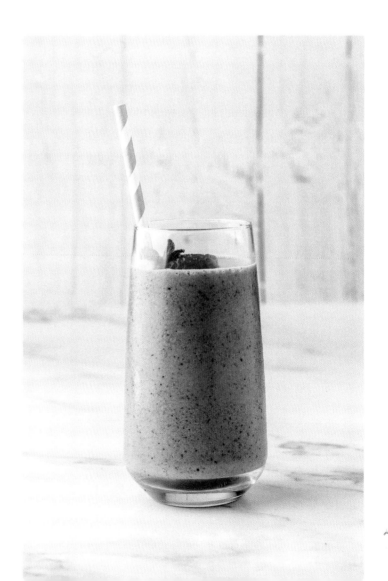

Apple & Avocado Smoothie

Serves: 1 | **Difficulty:** Easy | **Total time:** 5 min. | Suitable for vegetarians

....

Ingredients

200ml milk (any kind)

1 handful spinach leaves

1/2 small avocado, peeled and stoned

1 medium apple, cored and quartered

1 tsp honey (optional)

1/2 medium banana, cut into slices (the riper the better)

1 tsp ginger, finely grated

1/2 - 1 tbsp chia seeds

25g plain almonds

1 tbsp Greek yoghurt (optional – adds thickness and extra protein)

Handful of ice (if desired)

1. Add all ingredients together in a blender and blend until smooth.

Lemon & Ginger Zing Smoothie

Serves: 1 | **Difficulty:** Easy | **Total time:** 5 min. | Suitable for vegetarians

Ingredients

40g banana (best when frozen)

40g pineapple

Juice of 1/2 lemon (more if desired)

1/2 tbsp chia seeds (optional)

1 tbsp freshly grated ginger

200ml milk (any kind)

1 tsp honey (optional)

2 tbsp Greek yoghurt

Handful of ice (if desired)

1. Add all ingredients together in a blender and blend until smooth.

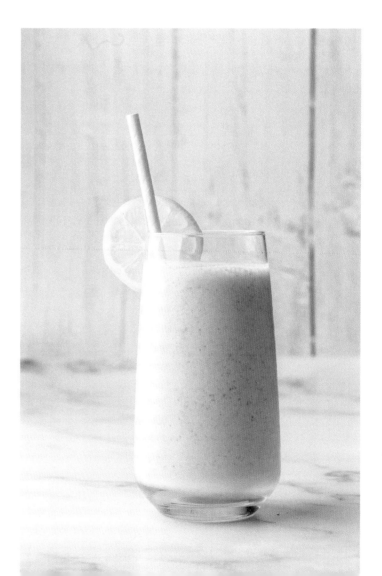

Mango & Passionfruit Delight

Serves: 1 | **Difficulty:** Easy | **Total time:** 5 min.

1. Add all ingredients together in a blender and blend until smooth.

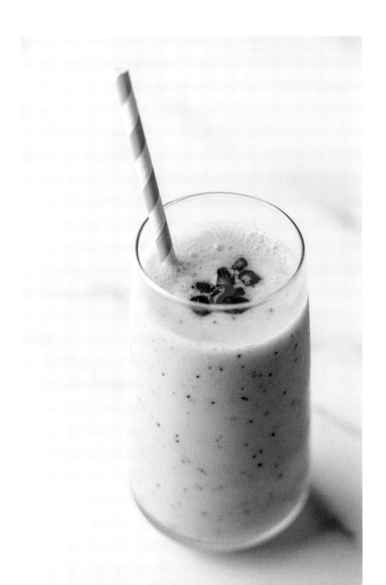

Ingredients

1 passion fruit (cut in half then scoop out the edible seeds and juicy inside fruit).

80g mango, cubed (frozen is best!)

1 tbsp Greek yoghurt

1 tbsp chia seeds

200ml coconut milk

Handful ice (if desired)

Peanut Butter & Banana Breakfast Smoothie

Serves: 1 | **Difficulty:** Easy | **Total time:** 5 min. | Suitable for vegetarians

Ingredients

1 large banana (the riper the better)

200ml milk (any kind)

1 tbsp Greek yoghurt

1 tbsp 100% natural peanut butter

1/2 tsp vanilla extract

Handful ice (if desired)

40g oats

1/2 tbsp cacao powder (optional)

1. Add all ingredients together in a blender and blend until smooth.

Cinnamon Kickstart

Serves: 1 | **Difficulty:** Easy | **Total time:** 5 min. | Suitable for vegetarians

Ingredients

5 pitted dates

1 tbsp pecans

200ml milk (almond milk is lovely with this recipe!)

1 tsp cinnamon

1 tsp vanilla extract

1 tbsp Greek yogurt

1/2 frozen banana

1 shot brewed coffee (chilled)

40g oats (optional)

Handful crushed ice

1. Add all ingredients together and blend until smooth.

Lunch

Lunches, for many people – including me, can be one of the harder meals to get creative with, especially if we have limited resources to keep the ingredients fresh or to heat up the food. That being said, I'd still much rather try and rustle up something of my own, rather than relying on shops or cafés to provide me with a suitable healthy meal on days when I'm not at home.

For this reason, I really like to make sure my lunches are well-planned for the week ahead to help me avoid looking for any shop-bought options. Spending a little time at the beginning of each week to plan and prepare for the meals you know you won't be at home for, can make a huge difference, not only to your health, but it can also save you money. That being said, it's really important that we don't become creatures of habit with our meals. Many people fall into the trap of eating the same thing for lunch every day when variety in our diet is so important. One of my favourite ways to make sure I have lots of variety when it comes to my lunches is to do regular batch cooking. Normally I like to make big batches of different soups and keep a supply of all of them in the freezer, packed in individual portions. This allows me to have a different kind of soup on a few days of the week, and I'll vary the rest of the week by having something else.

I have included a bunch of different recipes in here for you, to help inspire you to find heathy lunch ideas that can work for you. There's a whole mix of hot and cold ideas, so that you don't have to worry if you don't have a microwave for reheating.

One of the things I always preach about is just how useful it can be to invest in some decent containers or a good lunch bag that can help keep food cool. This means that you can take any meal or snack with you wherever you go. I'm usually the one who comes into work armed with different boxes of food to keep me going throughout the day. It's really a great way of helping you to stay on track with healthy eating.

Not only that, but why don't you take it in turns with a family member or colleague and do some lunch sharing? Find someone to take turns with on whose responsibility it is to make lunch on certain days of the week or maybe you could do alternate weeks in turn? This can make it more fun and can even save both of you some time and effort as well.

TUNA & BEAN PASTA SALAD WITH LEMON & OIL DRESSING

This one is great if you don't have a fridge to store it in as it can stay fresh for a few hours. It makes for a light and refreshing meal, yet it's still packed full of nutrients. This delicious option can help boost your energy levels and keep you going until dinner. (See page 183.)

SPICY BUTTERNUT SQUASH, COCONUT, RED LENTIL & GINGER SOUP

This has got to be one of my favourite soups and one which I'm often asked to make for Christmas Day because everyone likes it. That being said, it's a soup that I enjoy all year round and make often to have for lunch at work. It's so quick and easy to make and super filling, too, with a delicious, spicy kick. (See page 184.)

CARROT & BUTTER BEAN SOUP

I mentioned before that my mum is one of the people in my life who has played a huge part in developing my passion for food and cooking. My mum really is the Soup Queen, and there's always a bowl of soup ready for you whenever you pay her a visit. This next recipe is all down to her and it's one of my favourites – thanks, Mum, for letting me share it! It's so simple and quick to make and really delicious served with a warm buttered piece of bread. (See page 185.)

MANGO, ORANGE & AVOCADO BLACK BEAN SALAD

This plant-based recipe is so light and refreshing and one that takes little time to make. It can be stored at room temperature for a couple of hours, especially if it's kept in a cool bag, so this can be a good option if you don't have anywhere to keep your food at work. The flavour combination of the citrusy fruit and the fresh coriander go amazingly well together, and it's a favourite of mine to make, especially during the summer months. I often enjoy having a lighter meal for lunch at work, sometimes to help me avoid having that post-lunch slump. If you feel that you need to add in a little extra to this meal, it also goes great with some wholegrain rice tossed into it. (See page 186.)

TUNA & APPLE PITA

Minimal effort and time is required for this lunchtime choice, which means minimal washing up. These are just some of the reasons why I love making this for my lunch. I like to put together the filling the night before and just take it along with me in a separate container for lunch the next day. This means I can add the filling to the pita when I'm ready to eat it to stop it from making the pita bread soggy! (See page 187.)

CAJUN CHICKEN WRAP

This recipe is another one which is so quick and simple to make and can easily be prepped the night before to save you time. If I choose this, I like to take the fillings along with me separately and assemble them just before eating. This recipe is honestly so delicious and can also be a great for an evening meal. You can also easily double or even triple the ingredients if you're having friends over for a meal! (See page 188.)

PESTO BEAN PASTA

This is another healthy lunch option which is so simple and quick to make and contains ingredients that you probably already have in your kitchen. It is best eaten cold, and it's also a great one for whipping up the night before so that it's ready to grab and go from the fridge the next morning. (See page 189.)

CARROT, LEEK & TOMATO SOUP

I find soup so unbelievably comforting. There's really nothing better than a warm bowl of soup and having some freshly baked bread to go along with it. When I was in high school, I would often go visit my gran during my lunch break and I used to always sit and have a bowl of tomato soup with her. I think that's also why this is one of my favourite soup recipes, as it always reminds me of her. It's so simple to make and is packed full of vegetables and protein, making it far more nutritious compared to many of the shop-bought soups we see today. (See page 190.)

CURRIED PARSNIP & RED LENTIL SOUP

This is another one of the soups I make often and keep a ready supply of in my freezer. It's packed full of vegetables and contains a source of plant-based protein. This recipe makes 5-6 servings, so a few lunches (or dinners!) are prepared if you make a whole batch of this soup. (See page 191.)

SMOKED SALMON & CREAM CHEESE CRACKERS

Another time when plenty of containers comes in handy! I have this so often for lunch at work and spend just five minutes preparing it all the night before and putting the different ingredients in different containers ready to grab and go in the morning and then just assemble at lunch. Wonderfully easy to make, it is a super delicious, nourishing lunch, providing you with lots of protein, Omega-3 fats and a great source of calcium. (See page 192.)

BEETROOT & QUINOA FETA SALAD

Just the look of this salad is tempting! It's so bright and colourful, and the taste and texture combinations in this recipe are delicious. I absolutely love pomegranates, and since they're a colourful and healthy addition to most salads, it's a tasty fruit that I pick up often at the supermarkets. (See page 192.)

CHICKEN, COUSCOUS & CHICKPEA SALAD

This little recipe packs a protein punch with a delicious spicy kick. It's another recipe which is so full of flavour, packed with lots of nutrients yet simple and easy to make, containing a lot of ingredients that you will likely already have. This dish can also be made suitable for vegetarians or vegans with a few simple tweaks. It is just as lovely without the chicken, with the chickpeas still offering a good source of plant-based protein. It also goes great with some grilled tofu or tempeh instead. (See page 194.)

BAKED POTATO WITH PINEAPPLE & COTTAGE CHEESE

I always prefer baked potatoes made in the oven because I really think that it gives the potato that extra fluffy texture on the inside and a delicious, crispy skin on the outside. Rather than baking the whole potato in the microwave at work, often what I prefer to do is bake the potato in the oven at home the night before and just reheat it at lunch the next day in a microwave. Containers come in handy again for this recipe, so you can prepare the filling separately and put it all together just when you're ready to eat! This filling is also lovely with sweet potatoes, too. (See page 195.)

CHICKEN & HUMMUS CLUB SANDWICH

Who says homemade sandwiches have to be boring? How many times have you made a sandwich for lunch, took it out to eat and just thought, that doesn't look at all appetising? Forget the idea of having only ham and cheese and try out this delicious filling instead. It's also packed full of protein and healthy fats with a delicious homemade hummus. Sit back, enjoy, and fall in love with sandwiches again. (See page 196.)

LEMON & HONEY HALLOUMI & QUINOA SALAD

This salad just screams summer! It's so light and refreshing and so delicious that it also can be eaten at any time of the year. It's lovely for dinner as well, and if you're not a fan of halloumi, it's delicious with grilled chicken, tofu or feta cheese, too. (See page 197.)

Tuna & Bean Pasta Salad With Lemon & Oil Dressing

Serves: 1-2 | **Difficulty:** Easy | **Prep time:** 10 min. | **Cook time:** 10 min.

1. Cook the pasta as per package instructions.

2. In a large bowl, add the pasta and all the remaining ingredients.

3. Toss together, then serve.

Ingredients

75g uncooked wholegrain pasta

1/2 lemon juice + zest

Handful fresh parsley, finely chopped

5 cherry tomatoes

1/2 yellow pepper, diced

1/2 orange pepper, diced

1/2 red onion, diced

3 spring onions, finely chopped

1/2 tsp chilli flakes

100g can butter beans

Salt and pepper, to taste

Drizzle of extra virgin olive oil

30g Roasted Spicy Chickpeas (See my recipe in Healthy Snacks.)

140g tuna

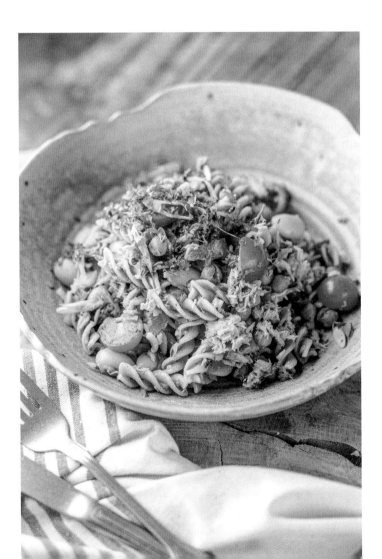

Spicy Butternut Squash, Coconut, Red Lentil & Ginger Soup

Serves: 5-6 | **Difficulty:** Easy | **Total time:** 50 min. | Suitable for vegetarians and vegans

Ingredients

1 tbsp olive oil

1 butternut squash, peeled, seeded and diced

3 garlic cloves, crushed

2 onions, diced

2 carrots, grated

1 thumb-sized piece of ginger, peeled and grated

1 red chilli, diced

900ml vegetable stock

100g red lentils

1 tin light coconut milk

1 tsp chopped coriander (optional for topping)

1 tsp chilli flakes (optional for topping)

1. Heat oil in a large pan and add butternut squash, garlic and onion.

2. Cook for 5 minutes, stirring regularly.

3. Add carrots, ginger and chilli and cook 3-5 minutes more, continuing to stir often.

4. Add vegetable stock and stir thoroughly.

5. Then add the lentils and coconut milk and stir to combine.

6. Bring the soup to boil, then lower to a simmer for 20 minutes.

7. Once the soup has finished cooking, blend with a hand blender or similar appliance until smooth.

8. Season with salt and pepper (to taste) and top with optional toppings, if desired.

9. This soup is delicious served with toasted rye bread.

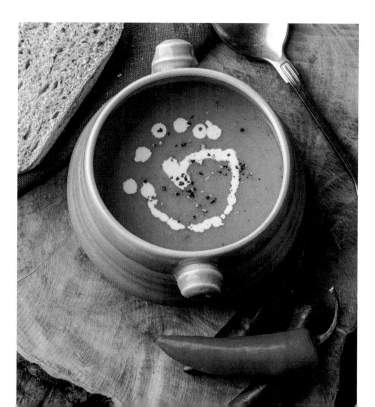

Carrot & Butter Bean Soup

Serves: 5-6 | **Difficulty:** Easy | **Total time:** 40 min. | Suitable for vegetarians and vegans

1. Soak the butter beans overnight in a bowl of fresh cold water, or as per package instructions. Make sure they are thoroughly rinsed in water afterwards.

2. Fill a large pot with approx. 2/3 water.

3. Add the stock cubes, onions, carrots and butter beans.

4. Bring to a boil and then simmer for 40-45 minutes until the butter beans are softened.

5. Season with salt and pepper, to taste.

6. Blend with a hand blender, if desired for a smoother texture.

7. Top with parsley to serve.

Ingredients

450g carrots, grated

450g onions, chopped

225g dried butter beans

3 stock cubes of your choice – I use chicken stock cubes for this recipe

Salt and pepper, to taste

Chopped fresh parsley, to taste

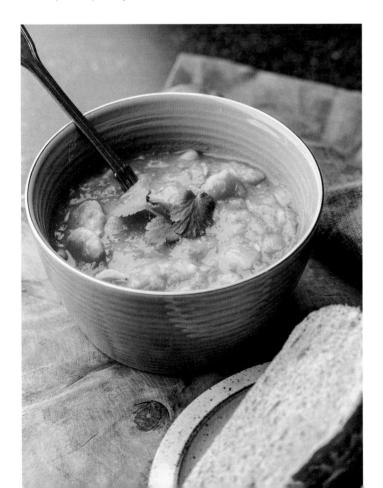

Mango, Orange & Avocado Black Bean Salad

Serves: 2 | **Difficulty:** Easy | **Total time:** 15 min. | Suitable for vegetarians and vegans

Ingredients

1 mango, peeled, stoned and diced

1/4 - 1/2 red onion, finely chopped

200g can black beans, drained and rinsed

Juice 1/2 orange

1-2 avocados, peeled, stoned and diced

1/2 - 1 tsp chilli flakes (or 1 fresh chilli, seeded and finely chopped)

3 spring onions, diced

1 handful of rocket leaves

1 red pepper, diced

Chopped fresh coriander, to taste

Salt and black pepper, to taste

1. Combine all ingredients in a large bowl and serve. Delicious served as a side salad or even with rice to make it a more balanced meal.

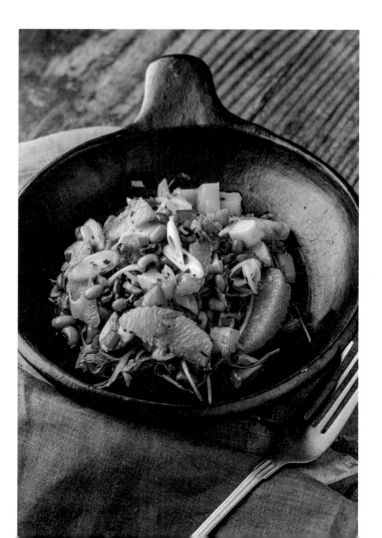

Tuna & Apple Pita

Serves: 1 | **Difficulty:** Easy | **Total time:** 10 min.

Ingredients

60g tinned tuna in spring water, drained

1/4 red onion, finely chopped

1 spring onions finely chopped

1/2 red apple, finely chopped

50g Greek yoghurt, or more to taste

Salt and pepper, to taste

Zest and juice of 1/2 lemon

1/4 tsp garlic powder

1/2 tsp dried parsley (optional)

1 small wholemeal pita bread

Small handful of mixed salad leaves or lettuce

1. Combine tuna, red onion, spring onions, apple, yoghurt, seasoning, lemon, garlic, and parsley.

2. Fill pita pocket with lettuce/salad leaves then add the tuna filling and enjoy!

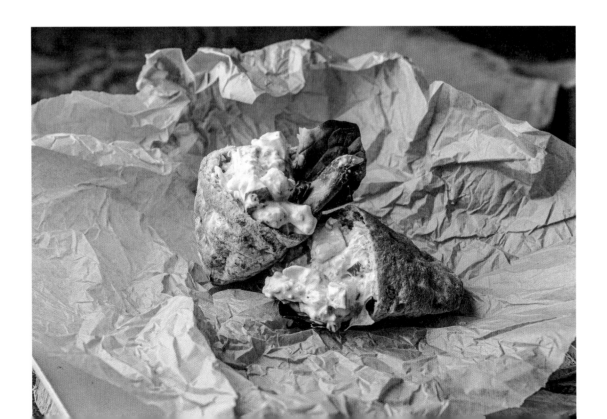

Cajun Chicken Wrap

Serves: 1 | **Difficulty:** Easy | **Total time:** 20 min.

Ingredients

100g chicken breasts, skin removed and cut into strips

1 garlic clove, crushed

Juice of 1 lime

2 tsp Cajun seasoning

1/2 tbsp. olive oil

1/2 avocado, diced

1/4 red onion, finely sliced

3 cherry tomatoes, finely diced

1/4 cucumber, diced

Pinch of chopped fresh coriander

1 wholemeal tortilla wrap

Salt and pepper to taste

10g low-fat cheddar cheese, grated (optional)

Small handful of lettuce or mixed salad leaves

1. In a large bowl, combine the chicken, garlic, 1/2 the lime juice and Cajun seasoning, and refrigerate for at least 10 minutes.

2. Heat the oil in a medium frying pan, over medium heat. Cook the chicken for approx.. 4-5 minutes until the chicken is cooked throughout. Place the chicken strips on some paper towels to drain any excess oil and set them aside to cool.

3. In a bowl, combine the avocado, red onion, tomatoes, cucumber and coriander with the remainder of the lime juice. Season this with salt and pepper, as desired.

4. To assemble, place the tortilla wrap on a flat work surface. Add lettuce/salad leaves to the middle of the wrap and top with the avocado mixture, then the chicken. Sprinkle with the grated cheese, then roll the wrap up and enjoy.

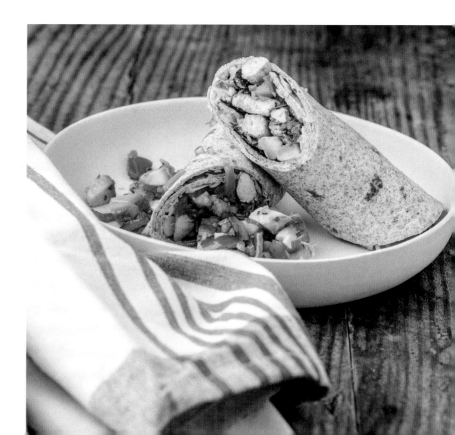

Pesto Bean Pasta

Serves: 2 | **Difficulty:** Easy | **Total time:** 25 min. | Suitable for vegetarians

....

Ingredients

150g uncooked, wholemeal pasta

1/2 tbsp - 1 tbsp reduced fat green pesto

200g black beans, drained and rinsed

8 cherry tomatoes, quartered

1/2 red pepper, finely chopped

2 tbsp sweet corn

4 spring onions, chopped

Salt and pepper, to taste

Grated parmesan, to taste (optional)

1/2 tsp chilli flakes (optional)

1/2 tbsp lemon juice (optional)

1. Cook the pasta according to the cooking instructions on the package.
2. In a large bowl, add the pasta, pesto, black beans cherry tomatoes, red pepper, sweet corn and spring onions. Gently mix all ingredients together so they have a coating of pesto.
3. Season with salt and pepper to taste.
4. Delicious served like this, but also lovely with an extra squeeze of lemon juice and a sprinkle of chilli flakes and parmesan.

Carrot, Leek & Tomato Soup

Serves: 5-6 | **Difficulty:** Easy | **Total time:** 40 min. | Suitable for vegetarians and vegans

Ingredients

25g butter (or vegan oil alternative)

1 large onion, finely chopped

450g carrots, finely diced

4 celery sticks, finely diced

225g medium leeks, trimmed and thinly sliced

400ml tomato passata/strained tomatoes

575ml vegetable stock

100g haricot beans

2 tsp Worcestershire sauce

Salt and black pepper to taste

Natural yoghurt, to garnish (optional)

Freshly chopped parsley, to garnish (optional)

Spring onions, finely chopped, to garnish (optional)

1. Melt the butter in a large, deep saucepan. Add the onion, carrots, celery and leeks and sauté over medium heat for approximately 5 minutes, until softened, not browned.

2. Pour in the passata/strained tomatoes, vegetable stock and haricot beans and stir thoroughly.

3. Add in the Worcestershire sauce and season to taste.

4. Bring to a boil, cover and then simmer for about 15-20 minutes until all the vegetables are tender.

5. Optional: Blend either half to all of the soup to your desired consistency.

6. Serve into bowls and garnish as desired, with a dollop of yoghurt and a sprinkle of spring onions and parsley.

Curried Parsnip & Red Lentil Soup

Serves: 5-6 | **Difficulty:** Easy | **Total time:** 60 min. | Suitable for vegetarians and vegans

1. Preheat oven to 160°C.

2. Take the finely sliced parsnips and pat them dry with a paper towel before drizzling over 1/2 tbsp oil.

3. Cover the parsnips with a dusting of cumin and season with salt and black pepper.

4. Place the parsnip slices on a baking tray covered in baking parchment and bake in the oven for approx. 20-25 minutes, until golden and crisp.

5. Meanwhile, in a large and deep saucepan, heat the remaining oil at medium heat.

6. Add the onion and sauté until the onion becomes transparent.

7. Add the potato and garlic and stir for a few more minutes.

8. Add the garam masala, coriander, turmeric and ginger and stir thoroughly.

9. Add the parsnips and sauté for a few minutes.

10. Add the vegetable stock, red lentils, bay leaves, salt and black pepper to taste.

11. Bring to a boil, cover and then simmer for approx. 20 minutes until the parsnips are tender.

12. Blend in an electric blender until smooth.

13. Serve in a warm bowl and top with crème fraiche, chilli flakes, the parsnip crisps from the oven and some fresh coriander.

Ingredients

750g parsnips, peeled with 100g finely sliced and 650g roughly chopped

1 1/2 tbsp olive oil

1/4 tsp ground cumin

1 brown onion, finely chopped

1 medium potato, peeled and chopped

1 garlic clove, crushed

1 tsp garam masala

1 tsp dried, ground coriander

1/4 tsp turmeric

1 1/2 tsp ground or fresh ginger (peeled and finely grated)

1200ml vegetable stock

Salt and black pepper, to taste

100g red lentils

2 bay leaves

Sprinkle of chilli flakes to garnish (optional)

Fresh coriander leaves, to garnish

Crème fraiche to garnish

Smoked Salmon & Cream Cheese Crackers

Serves: 1 | **Difficulty:** Easy | **Total time:** 10 min.

Ingredients

2 tbsp low-fat cream cheese

1/4 tsp garlic powder

Zest and juice of 1/2 lemon

Salt and black pepper, to taste

4 wholegrain crackers

50g smoked salmon

1/2 tsp dried dill

1/4 red onion, finely chopped

Handful of rocket leaves

1. In a bowl, combine the cream cheese, garlic powder, lemon zest and juice.

2. Season with sea salt and black pepper to taste.

3. Spread a thin layer on each cracker and top with some rocket leaves.

4. Divide the smoked salmon evenly over the crackers and garnish with dill, red onion, extra salt and pepper as desired and add some extra lemon juice to taste.

Beetroot & Quinoa Feta Salad

Serves: 2 | **Difficulty:** Easy | **Total time:** 40 min.

Ingredients

2 baby corn ears, cut into slices

4 asparagus stalks, woody ends removed

1 red pepper, cored, seeded and diced

1/2 tbsp olive oil

150g sweet potato, chopped into small cubes

Sea salt and black pepper, to taste

75g quinoa, rinsed

150ml vegetable stock

80g pomegranate

1 large cooked beetroot, cut into wedges

Handful of rocket leaves

1 tbsp lemon juice

50g feta cheese, crumbled

1/2 tbsp pumpkin seeds

1. Preheat oven grill/broiler to medium heat.

2. Place the corn, asparagus and pepper in an oven-proof dish and add a drizzle of olive oil. Broil underneath the grill until vegetables are lightly browned. Remove from the heat and leave aside to cool.

3. Preheat oven to 180°C.

4. Line a roasting pan with baking parchment and add the sweet potato. Drizzle a small amount of oil over the sweet potato and season well with salt and black pepper. Put in the oven and roast for approx. 20 minutes.

5. Meanwhile, cook the quinoa as per package instructions using the vegetable stock.

6. Chop the asparagus and red pepper into smaller slices, if desired, and add to a large bowl.

7. Add the quinoa and pomegranate to the bowl and mix well.

8. Once the sweet potato has cooked, add it and the beetroot to the bowl and stir thoroughly.

9. Add lemon juice and rocket leaves and toss all the ingredients together.

10. Spoon the salad onto a serving dish and top with crumbled feta and pumpkin seeds.

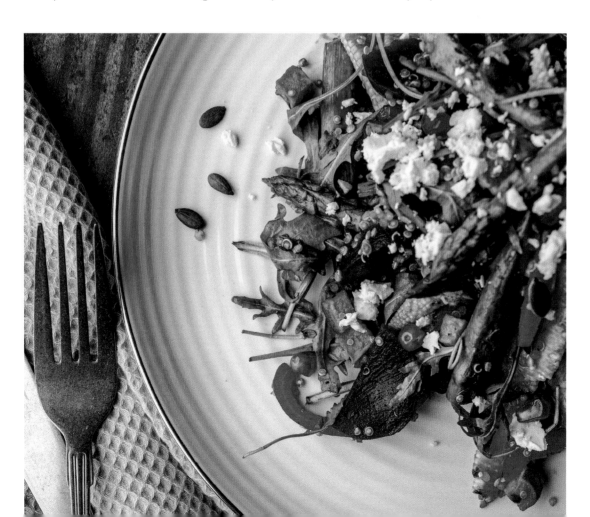

Chicken, Couscous & Chickpea Salad

Serves: 2 | **Difficulty:** Easy | **Total time:** 20 min.

Ingredients

100g couscous

100ml vegetable stock

1 tbsp olive oil

Juice and zest 1/2 lime

1/2 tbsp harissa paste (Tunisian hot chilli pepper paste – this is very spicy!)

75g spicy chickpeas (See my snack recipe section.)

80g cooked chicken breast, chopped

80g cucumber, chopped

1 carrot, thinly sliced or grated

80g cherry tomatoes, quartered

1/2 small red onion, finely chopped

1 tbsp mixed freshly chopped mint, basil and parsley

1. Put the couscous in a bowl and pour the boiling stock over it. Set aside for 5 minutes until most or all of the stock has been absorbed.

2. In a mug or separate bowl, combine the oil, lime juice and harissa paste with a fork and set aside.

3. Break up the couscous with a fork so it's light and fluffy.

4. In a large bowl, combine the couscous, chickpeas, chicken, cucumber, carrot, tomatoes, onion and herbs to the couscous and stir to combine.

5. Season with salt and pepper to taste.

6. Serve the chicken and couscous mix on a bed of rocket and drizzle the harissa sauce over to taste.

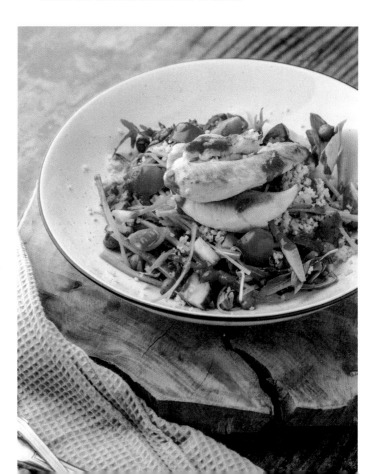

Baked Potato With Pineapple & Cottage Cheese

Serves: 1 | **Difficulty:** Easy | **Total time:** 70 min.

1. Preheat oven to 180°C.

2. Place the potato on a baking tray and drizzle a little olive oil over the potato and season with salt and pepper, to taste.

3. Place the potato in the middle of the oven and bake for approx. 1 hour until skin is crispy and a knife pierces through with ease.

4. Meanwhile, mix together the cottage cheese, spring onions, pineapple, cucumber and dill in a bowl and then season to taste with sea salt and black pepper.

5. Cut the potato open and fill the inside with the cottage cheese filling.

Ingredients

1 medium baking potato, pierced all over with a fork

120g low-fat cottage cheese

2 spring onions, finely chopped

1 pineapple ring, finely chopped

1/2 cucumber, finely chopped

1/2 tsp dried dill

Salt and black pepper, to taste

Chicken & Hummus Club Sandwich

Serves: 1 | **Difficulty:** Easy | **Total time:** 15 min.

Ingredients

2 slices wholegrain bread

3 tbsp of homemade lemon and coriander hummus (See my Dips and Spreads recipe section.)

Handful of rocket leaves

1/2 avocado, peeled, stoned and sliced

80g cooked breast chicken, sliced

4 cherry tomatoes, quartered

Salt and pepper to taste

1. Toast the bread (as desired).

2. Spread the homemade hummus evenly onto one side of each slice of bread.

3. Layer on the rocket, avocado, chicken breast and tomato.

4. Season as desired.

5. op with the other slice of toast and cut the sandwich into quarters.

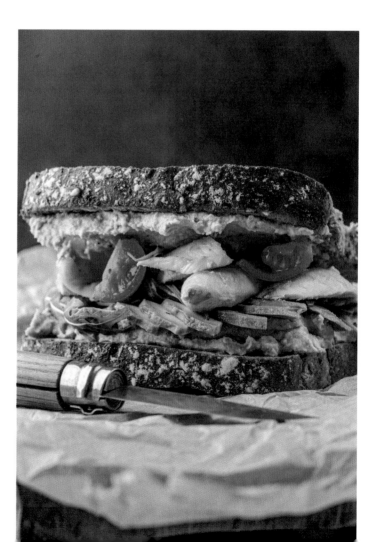

Lemon & Honey Halloumi & Quinoa Salad

Serves: 2 | **Difficulty:** Easy | **Total time:** 15 min.

1. Preheat oven grill to medium heat.

2. Drain the cooked quinoa and place in a large bowl. Using a fork, break up the quinoa so it's light and fluffy. Set aside.

3. Grill the halloumi slices for 4-5 minutes until golden brown.

4. In a small bowl, combine the olive oil, lemon juice, honey and garlic. Combine until smooth. Season to taste.

5. Add peas, spring onions, cherry tomatoes, chopped yellow pepper and fresh coriander to the bowl with the quinoa and stir until all the ingredients are well mixed.

6. Pour the lemon dressing over the salad and toss thoroughly.

7. Serve on two separate plates and top with the halloumi cheese and a sprinkle of mixed seeds.

Ingredients

120g quinoa, cooked as per package instructions

80g reduced fat halloumi cheese

1 tbsp olive oil

Juice of 1 lemon

1 tsp honey

1 garlic clove, crushed

Sea salt and black pepper, to taste

75g cooked peas

3 spring onions, thinly sliced

8 cherry tomatoes, quartered

1 yellow pepper, chopped

10g fresh coriander, finely chopped

1 tbsp mixed seeds

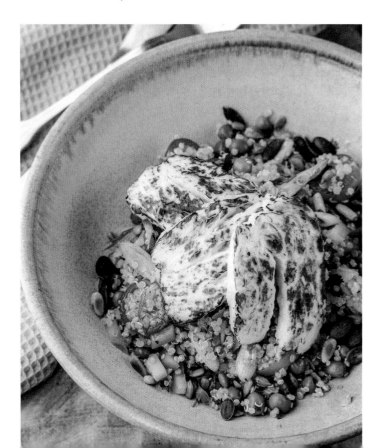

Dinner

At the end of a busy day, there's nothing better than coming home and sitting down to enjoy a delicious meal. If you're anything like me, although I really love to cook, my motivation to get in the kitchen in the evening is usually pretty low. This is why I am a lover of batch cooking. I love spending a bit of time at the weekend making a few big batches of different foods, e.g. bolognese, chilli, curry, soups, stews, etc. so that I always have a supply of some hearty, nourishing meals in my freezer to help me out on nights I can't be bothered with cooking.

Another useful tip I can give you when it comes to making dinners is to make double the amount and save the extra for lunch the next day. This can save you prepping another food item for lunch in the evening if you haven't got anything else ready for the next day!

I have included some of my favourite healthy dinner recipes here for you. There are loads that are suitable for batch cooking at the weekend, so you'll be ready and prepared for the working week ahead, or some of which can be rustled up in half an hour after a long day. There are also some lovely recipes which are great for those weekend days when you may have a little extra time to spend in the kitchen to create something really delicious for family and friends.

LENTIL & CHICKPEA CURRY

This has to be one of my all-time favourite plant-based meals, and one which I regularly make at the weekend. It's super filling, provides lots of great fibre to support our gut health and contains great sources of plant-based protein. This recipe can also be easily doubled if you want to make a bigger batch. (See page 203.)

GARLIC & LIME SEABASS WITH PECAN & ROSEMARY SWEET POTATO MASH

This recipe just needs a little bit of sensible timing to get it all ready at the same time, but otherwise, it is pretty simple to make. The sweet potato mash is given a lovely creamy texture, thanks to the butter and cheese, and made even more delicious served up with the maple and rosemary all mixed through it, too.

Seabass is a lovely fish, but I know it's not always easy to get all year round. If you struggle to find it at your supermarket or fish monger, this recipe also goes well with any other white fish and even salmon, too. What I love about this recipe is that just a tiny splash of lime and a bit of garlic goes a long way, giving white fish so much flavour. Keeping the fish loosely parcelled up in the baking foil during baking can also help to keep it nice and juicy and prevents the fish from drying out. (See page 204.)

PESTO & MOZZARELLA CHICKEN WITH HONEY & ROSEMARY SWEET POTATO MASH, BROCCOLI & FINE GREEN BEANS

Meat, potatoes and vegetables. This is often the make-up of a traditional dinner here in the UK – along with a huge serving of gravy. Don't get me wrong, this type of meal can be lovely and something I really enjoy having on a Sunday with my family. However, I've mixed it up a little with this recipe and added in some different ingredients to jazz up this UK favourite. (See page 206.)

CHILLI CON CARNE

I've mentioned before that I absolutely love Mexican food and chilli con carne has to really be up there in my top 5 favourite meals of all time. Chilli was made really often when I was a kid, and it's my dad's speciality dish to make. I get my love of Mexican and spicy food from my dad. His recipe is amazing, and we would always enjoy it with extra jalapenos and some garlic bread, too. This is my own version of a delicious chilli, packed with extra beans for an extra source of fibre and plant-based protein. I honestly find it so tasty, and it's great served with so many different things, such as traditional rice, or with tortilla chips if you want to make chilli nachos, stuffed into a baked potato and it also goes great with pasta! This is a staple dish I can guarantee you is in my freezer most weeks. A great source of protein, both animal and plant-based, packed full of vegetables and high in iron and fibre. This is a great meal to make if you have family and friends coming over as the quantities are very easily doubled and you can prepare it in advance, which means minimal time and stress in the kitchen when you've got company! I should say, too, you haven't misread the addition of a teaspoon of cinnamon in this recipe. It adds such a delicious, subtle flavour – don't leave it out! (See page 208.)

SPICY CHICKEN, TOMATO & RED PEPPER RISOTTO

Just wait until you have tried this one! I know so many people that struggle to get the right texture when making risotto – you don't want it too runny, but you also don't want it to dry out and be too thick either. This fool-proof recipe will make sure you get it right every time. The flavour of this is amazing and it takes just about 10 minutes to prepare before you can leave it to cook in the oven for a while, allowing you to do other things! (See page 210.)

TROPICAL JERK CHICKEN WITH COCONUT, PEA & BLACK BEAN RICE

This Jamaican-inspired recipe takes a little bit of extra time in the kitchen, but the end result is honestly worth the extra effort. The use of chicken thighs in this recipe makes it super juicy and tasty, but if you're not a fan of this cut of meat, you can also use chicken breasts, too. The spices and herbs used are the perfect balance of spicy heat as well as sweet and savoury and make for a truly delicious dish. (See page 212.)

HONEY, GARLIC & CHILLI SALMON

The ingredients in this recipe make a delicious sticky and sweet sauce which goes extremely well with salmon. It's super simple to make, and you'll also probably have a lot of the ingredients in your cupboard already. I love to serve this either with some rice or potatoes and some fresh vegetables, or it's really nice as part of a stir fry, too. (See page 214.)

KING PRAWN FRIED RICE

Super simple, super tasty and super delicious with minimal washing up. Another win-win! You should be trying to get a wide variety of protein sources in your diet, but if king prawns aren't your thing, chicken or tofu works great in this recipe, too. (See page 215.)

SPLIT PEA & POMEGRANATE SALAD

This eastern Mediterranean-inspired salad is full of fresh flavours such as mint, lemon and fresh parsley, and the sumac gives it a delicious, exotic twist. I love to let the bulgur wheat marinate for as long as possible, to let the flavours soak right in. This dish is packed full of plant-based protein and contains lots of vitamins and minerals, making it a really nutritious meal. It's also keeps well in the fridge and can also be enjoyed the next day, served cold for a lovely, light lunch. It can be made with some garlic mixed into it, too, and you can also use couscous instead of bulgur wheat, if you wish. (See page 216.)

SEABASS WITH BLACK RICE & MANGO SALSA

This simple dish is one that I often go to when I'm trying to impress my guests. If I can get my hands on some black rice, the colours of this dish are fantastic. That being said, it goes just as well served with some wholegrain rice or even homemade sweet potato fries. The mango salsa served with this recipe goes with pretty much any white fish as a really delicious and refreshing dressing, so don't worry if you can't get your hands on some seabass. (See page 217.)

GOATS CHEESE & WALDORF SALAD

This is a light salad suitable for both lunch and dinner. The dressing is made from yoghurt instead of mayonnaise, lowering the saturated-fat content, as well as giving you an extra source of protein and calcium. Walnuts are often the nut included in Waldorf salads, but you can mix in whatever nuts you like, and the salad also goes lovely with some halloumi or feta cheese, too, if you prefer. (See page 218.)

VEGGIE TACOS

Tacos are really one of my all-time favourite dinners. We often have 'taco night' in our family, and when we do, it's an absolute feast. Normally we use homemade beef bolognese in our tacos which is a personal favourite, but I also love having a plant-based version of this delicious dish, too. This is great if you have friends coming over for an evening. I love to make a bunch of different dips as well, like my avocado salsa and spicy tomato salsa, and just let everyone dig in and make their own tacos! (See page 219.)

CHICKEN & ORANGE SALAD

You'll find this a zesty, summery salad which is great for both lunch and dinner. It's really light and refreshing and uses a lot of basic ingredients that you'll likely already have in your kitchen. The flaked almonds add something special to the dish, packing in extra protein and healthy fats, as well as adding a delicious crunch! (See page 220.)

STICKY STEAK STIR FRY

Doesn't everyone love stir fry? They're a tasty way of adding lots of vegetables to your meal, they're cheaper and healthier than a take-away, and they're a great way of using up a lot of veg in your fridge. Not only that, but they're a simple and quick dinner that can be ready in as little as 20 minutes. This recipe is one of my best-loved ways to make a stir fry, which provides a great source of iron, but you can easily make your own stir fry by using other vegetables that you prefer, or by using different meats or plant-based protein – you can rarely go wrong! (See page 222.)

SPAGHETTI WITH TUNA, OLIVES & CAPERS

Here is yet another recipe which you'll likely have the majority of the ingredients for in your kitchen cupboards already. It's super light and super easy to make, but also super-filling, giving you a great source of protein and Omega-3 fats. (See page 223.)

QUICK & EASY HOMEMADE PIZZA BASE

Have you ever wondered how you can use up some leftover tortilla wraps? Use them as a pizza base! Don't get me wrong, if I had the time and the culinary skills to make my own pizza dough I would, but I've tried before and I have never managed to get it right, so I've decided that I'll just leave it to the experts. This recipe gives you an idea on how to make the base and the tomato sauce, but it leaves it open for you to add on whatever toppings you like, so be creative! My favourite is mozzarella, red onion, fresh basil and a drizzle of balsamic dressing. (See page 224.)

Lentil & Chickpea Curry

Serves: 2 | **Difficulty:** Easy | **Prep time:** 20 min. | **Cook time:** 20-25 min. | Suitable for vegetarians and vegans

1. Heat the olive oil in a deep saucepan over medium heat

2. Add onion, garlic, celery, green pepper, and chilli and cook gently for approx. 8-10 minutes or until the vegetables have started to soften.

3. Add the garam masala, cumin, and dried coriander and cook for 2-3 minutes more, stirring often.

4. Add the tomato puree, vegetable stock, tomato passata, lentils, coconut milk, and chickpeas to the saucepan.

5. Bring all of the ingredients to a boil then reduce the heat, cover and simmer for approx. 20-25 minutes, until lentils are soft and the sauce has thickened. During the last few minutes of cooking, add the chopped spinach and stir well.

6. Season to taste.

7. Meanwhile, cook the rice as per package instructions.

8. Serve the curry on a bed of the wholegrain rice and enjoy!

» *Option:*

This is also delicious served with naan bread.

Ingredients

1/2 tbsp. olive oil

1/2 brown onion, diced

1 garlic clove, crushed

1 celery stalk, diced

1 green pepper, diced

1-2 fresh chilli, finely diced (2 chillies if you like an extra spicy kick!)

1 tsp garam masala

1/2 tsp cumin

1/2 tsp dried coriander

1 tbsp tomato puree

350ml vegetable stock

200g fine tomato passata/strained tomatoes

75g red lentils

200ml light/reduced fat coconut milk

200g chickpeas, drained and rinsed

2-3 handfuls spinach, finely chopped

Salt and pepper, to taste

150g uncooked wholegrain rice

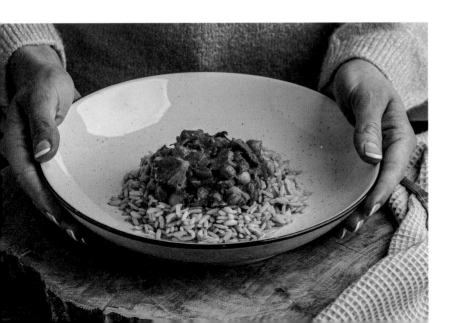

Garlic & Lime Seabass With Pecan & Rosemary Sweet Potato Mash

Serves: 2 | **Difficulty:** Moderate | **Prep time:** 15 min. | **Cook time:** 20 min.

Ingredients

2 seabass fillets

Juice of 1 lime

1 clove garlic, crushed

Salt and pepper

1 tsp butter

1 handful of fresh coriander, chopped finely

» *Sweet Potato Mash*

2 small sweet potatoes, peeled and diced

1/3 cup pecan pieces

1 tbsp olive oil

1/2 tsp chilli powder

1/2 tsp rosemary

1/2 - 1 tbsp butter

15g grated cheddar cheese

1/2 tbsp maple syrup

Sea salt and black pepper, to taste

» *To serve:* vegetables of your choice.

1. Preheat oven to 220°C.
2. Place the fish on a piece of aluminium foil on a baking tray and top each fish with approx. 1/2 tsp butter.
3. Cover the fish with half of the lime juice, add the crushed garlic and season with salt and pepper.
4. Loosely wrap the fish into a parcel with the foil and place the fish in the oven, baking for approx. 15 minutes.

5. In meantime, place the sweet potatoes into a medium pot and cover with water. Bring the water to a boil and then simmer for approx. 15 minutes until the potatoes are soft.

6. In the meantime, while the fish and the potatoes are cooking, line a baking tray with baking parchment and spread the pecans out all over the baking tray.

7. Drizzle the pecans with oil, chilli powder, rosemary, and salt and black pepper.

8. Roast the pecans in the oven for approx. 2-3 minutes. Their aroma should be fragrant. Be careful, they can burn quickly if not watched very closely. Take out and set aside.

9. Take the seabass fillets out of the oven after 15 minutes. Uncover them, top with the remaining lime juice, and add the coriander. Parcel up the fish again and bake for 10 minutes more (or until the end of the suggested cooking time as instructed on the package). The fish will be ready when the flesh flakes easily with a fork.

10. Once the potatoes are cooked, drain them and put them back in the pot. Add the butter, cheese, maple syrup, and salt and pepper and then mash together well.

11. Serve the sweet potatoes topped with the roasted pecans, alongside the seabass fillets and vegetables of your choice.

Pesto & Mozzarella Chicken With Honey & Rosemary Sweet Potato Mash, Broccoli & Fine Green Beans

Serves: 2 | **Difficulty:** Moderate | **Total time:** 30 min.

Ingredients

2 chicken breasts

3-4 tsp reduced fat green pesto

2 thin slices mozzarella

100ml tomato passata/strained tomatoes

1 tsp mixed Italian herbs

1 tsp oregano

Salt and pepper, to taste

2 small sweet potatoes, coarsely chopped

1 tsp butter

50ml milk

2 tbsp honey

2 tsp dried rosemary (optional)

40g fine green beans

40g broccoli

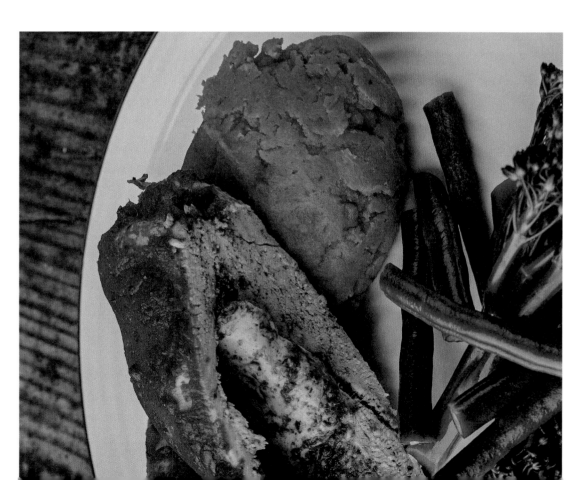

1. Preheat oven to 200°C.

2. Slice the chicken lengthways, but not all the way through, so the chicken is still in one piece at one end (so it opens like a book).

3. On the inside of the chicken breasts, cover each side with a thin layer of the pesto.

4. Place a slice of mozzarella inside each chicken breast and close it, encasing the pesto and mozzarella inside.

5. In a bowl, combine the tomato passata with the mixed herbs, oregano and salt and pepper.

6. Place the chicken breasts in an oven dish and spread the passata sauce evenly all over the chicken breasts.

7. Bake in the centre of the oven for approx. 25 minutes, until the chicken is thoroughly cooked.

8. In the meantime, put the sweet potatoes in a medium pot and cover with water. Bring the water to a boil and then simmer for approx. 15 minutes until the potatoes are soft.

9. At the same time, cook the fine green beans and broccoli according to instructions.

10. Once the potatoes are ready, drain them and put them back in the same pot. Add the butter, honey, rosemary, salt and black pepper and mash them all together.

11. Serve the mozzarella and pesto chicken on a bed of the sweet potato mash with a side of the vegetables. Add extra seasoning as desired.

Chilli Con Carne

Serves: 4 | **Difficulty:** Easy | **Total time:** 50 min. | Great for freezing

....

Ingredients

1 tbsp olive oil

1 large onion, finely chopped

2 garlic clove, crushed

1-2 red bell peppers, finely chopped

2 celery stalk, finely chopped

1-2 fresh chilli peppers, seeded and finely chopped (add more depending on taste preference)

1 tsp cayenne pepper

1 tsp cumin

1 tsp paprika

1 tsp cinnamon

1 tsp dried coriander

1 tsp chilli powder (for an extra chilli kick!)

400g lean minced beef

300ml beef stock

400g tomato passata

1 tbsp tomato puree

Salt and pepper, to taste

400g tin red kidney beans, drained and rinsed

200g black beans, drained and rinsed

300g uncooked brown rice

Salt and pepper to taste

Low-fat Greek or natural yoghurt to taste (optional)

1. Put a large, deep pot over medium heat and add the olive oil.

2. Add the onion and cook for approx. 3-5 minutes until the onion is transparent.

3. Add the garlic, red bell peppers, celery and fresh chilli peppers, along with cayenne pepper, cumin, paprika, cinnamon, coriander and chilli powder, if preferred. Stir well and leave to cook for another few minutes.

4. Turn the heat up a little and add the lean minced beef. Stir thoroughly and ensure the mince is broken up well into small pieces. Continue to cook until there are no more pink ground beef pieces in the pot.

5. Add 300ml beef stock and stir well.

6. Add the tomato passata, salt and pepper and the tomato puree.

7. Bring it to a boil, reduce the heat and then simmer for approx. 20 minutes, stirring occasionally. The mixture should be thick, moist and juicy.

8. Add the kidney beans and black beans and simmer again for another 10 minutes.

9. Leave to stand in the pot for approx. 10 minutes. While doing so, cook the rice as per package instructions.

10. Serve the chilli on top of the rice with an extra sprinkle of the fresh chilli and yoghurt, if desired.

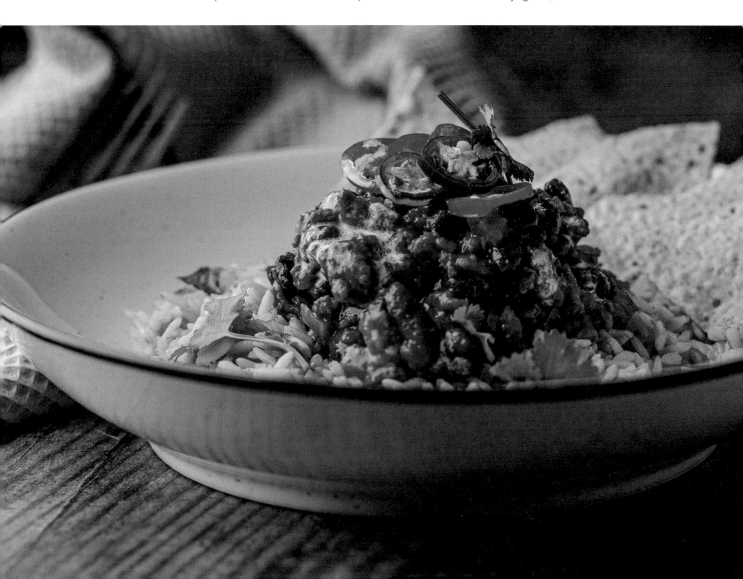

Spicy Chicken, Tomato & Red Pepper Risotto

Serves: 2-3 | **Difficulty:** Easy | **Prep time:** 10 min. | **Cook time:** 35-40 min.

Ingredients

300g chicken, diced

1 tbsp olive oil

1 onion, diced

1 garlic clove

300g risotto rice

2 red bell peppers, chopped

1-2 fresh chillies, finely diced

1 tsp dried parsley

400ml tomato passata/strained tomatoes

6 piccolo tomatoes, halved

450-500ml chicken or vegetable stock

Salt and pepper, to taste

Parmesan shavings, to taste

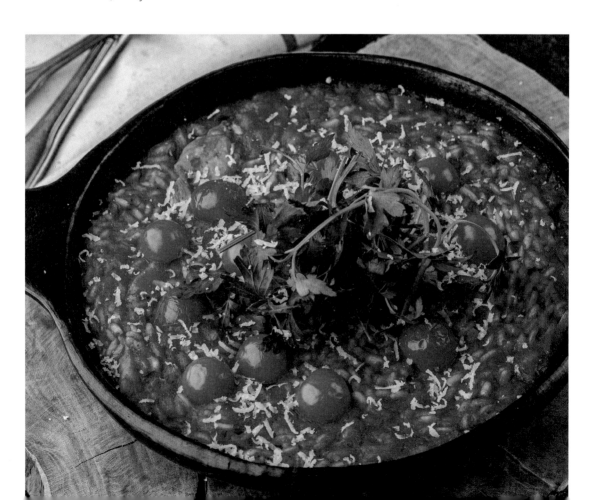

1. Preheat oven to 200°C.

2. Add 1/2 tbsp oil to a wok/frying pan and set at medium heat.

3. Add the chicken and stir fry it until it is cooked through. Take the chicken out and lay it on some paper towels to drain away any excess oil and set aside.

4. Set a large pot over medium heat and add 1/2 tbsp oil. Add the garlic and onion and stir fry for a few minutes until the onion has become transparent.

5. Add the risotto rice and cook for a few more minutes, stirring regularly.

6. Add chicken, bell peppers, chillies, and dried parsley, followed by the tomato passata, stock then salt and pepper. Stir thoroughly.

7. Place the mixture into an oven-proof dish and top with the tomatoes.

8. Cover the dish with aluminium foil and bake for approx. 35-40 minutes until piping hot and the sauce is nice and creamy.

9. Take the dish out of the oven and top the risotto with parmesan shavings before serving.

Tropical Jerk Chicken With Coconut, Pea & Black Bean Rice

Serves: 2 | **Difficulty:** Medium | **Total time:** 1 hr. 45 min

Ingredients

2 chicken thighs

2 tinned pineapple rings

100mls pineapple juice (from tin)

8 spring onions, chopped (4 for marinade, 4 for rice)

1 garlic clove, crushed

Small piece of ginger, peeled and grated

1/4 - 1/2 onion, finely chopped

2 red chillies – chopped

3/4 tsp dried thyme

Juice of 1 lime

1 tbsp soy sauce

1 tbsp extra virgin olive oil

3/4 tsp cinnamon

3/4 tsp nutmeg

1 tsp all spice

Black pepper, to taste

Optional: 1 tsp brown sugar

» *Rice*

1/2 can light coconut milk (200ml)

400ml water

Salt, to taste

150g uncooked rice

200g can black beans, drained and rinsed

3 tbsp garden peas

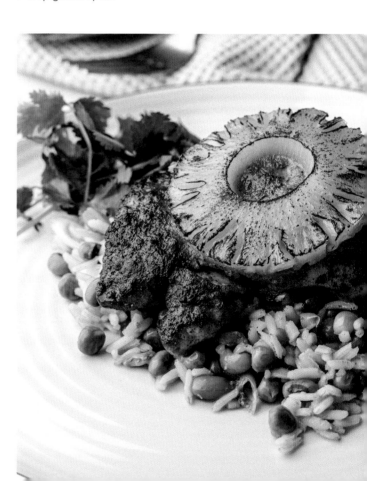

1. Place two chicken thighs on a baking tray and pour the pineapple juice over them.

2. If using a blender, add 4 spring onions, garlic, ginger, onion, red chilli, thyme, 1/2 lime juice, soy sauce, olive oil, cinnamon, nutmeg, all spice, and black pepper and then blend to form a puree. If a blender is not available, just chop the vegetables as finely as possible and mix everything together by hand.

3. Spoon the blended puree over the chicken thighs and marinate in the fridge for at least 1 hour.

4. Heat the oven to 160°C.

5. Top each of the chicken thighs with a pineapple ring.

6. Optional: add a sprinkle of brown sugar to the pineapple rings to caramelise in the oven.

7. Bake the chicken in oven for 45 min, until chicken is cooked through.

8. Meanwhile, in a medium pot, combine coconut milk, water and salt. Add the rice to the pot and cook the rice as per package instructions.

9. Meanwhile, cook the black beans and peas as per package instructions.

10. When the rice is cooked, drain it and put it into a bowl. Add the remaining lime juice and mix through.

11. Add the black beans and peas to the rice along with the remaining spring onions and combine. Season to taste.

12. Serve the chicken on a bed of the coconut rice.

Honey, Garlic & Chilli Salmon

Serves: 2 | **Difficulty:** Easy | **Total time:** 15 min.

Ingredients

1 salmon fillet

1/2 tsp paprika

Salt and black pepper, to taste

1 tbsp butter

1 garlic clove, crushed

1-2 tbsp honey

1/2 tbsp water

1 tsp soy sauce

Juice 1/2 lemon

1/2 tsp chilli flakes

1. Heat the oven grill/broiler.

2. Place the salmon on a plate and season with salt, pepper and paprika and set aside.

3. In medium pan, melt the butter over low heat.

4. Add the garlic and cook for 1-2 minutes until fragrant.

5. Add honey, water, soy sauce, lemon juice, and chilli flakes and mix well.

6. Add the salmon to a frying or griddle pan, skin side down. Cook at medium-high heat until golden for approx. 3-4 minutes, occasionally basting the top of the salmon in the sauce.

7. Place the pan under the grill and broil the salmon for approx. 5-6 more minutes until it is cooked through. It should flake easily with a fork.

8. Season with more lemon juice if desired and serve with potatoes or rice and your choice of vegetables.

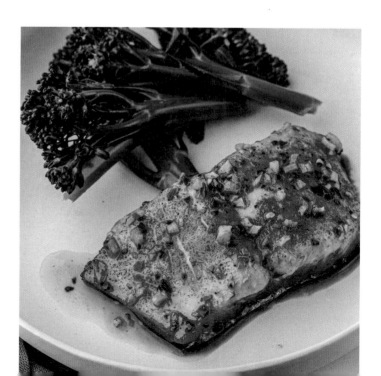

King Prawn Fried Rice

Serves: 1 | **Difficulty:** Easy | **Total time:** 15 min.

1. Cook the rice as per package instructions and set aside.

2. Heat the oil in a non-stick frying pan. Add onion and garlic and cook for a few minutes until the onion becomes transparent.

3. Add the cooked rice and cook through for another 1-2 minutes.

4. Push the rice to one side of the pan and add the beaten egg. Scramble the egg for a minute or two, continuously stirring, then combine the egg and rice together.

5. Add the spring onions, baby corn cobs and pea pods and cook for a few more minutes.

6. Add the king prawns, soy sauce, honey, lemon juice, and zest and stir thoroughly. Cook for another minute or two to heat through.

7. Serve in two bowls and top with coriander. Add extra soy sauce, if desired.

Ingredients

150g uncooked wholegrain rice

2 tbsp olive oil

1 red onion

1 garlic clove, crushed

1 egg, beaten

4 spring onions, finely chopped

2 baby corn cobs, chopped

100g mangetout/snow peas

10 large king prawns

1 tbsp light soy sauce

1/2 tbsp honey

Zest and juice of 1 lemon

2 tbsp chopped coriander

Split Pea & Pomegranate Salad

Serves: 1-2 | **Difficulty:** Easy | **Total time:** 1 hr. | Suitable for vegetarians and vegans

Ingredients

50g Bulgur wheat

30g yellow split peas

Small handful of fresh flat-leafed parsley, roughly chopped

5 cherry tomatoes, quartered

Small handful fresh mint leaves

2 spring onions, thinly chopped

1/2 orange bell pepper, finely sliced

1/2 tbsp olive oil

Juice and zest of 1/2 lemon

1/2 tsp sumac

20g pomegranate

Salt and pepper, to taste

1. In a bowl, add the bulgur wheat and cover with boiling water. Allow the bulgur wheat to expand, then leave it to cool for approx. 30 minutes.

2. In a saucepan, add the yellow split peas. Cover with plenty of water, bring to a boil, cover, then simmer for approx. 25 minutes, until peas are tender.

3. Meanwhile, add the parsley, tomatoes, mint leaves, spring onion and bell pepper to a large bowl and mix together.

4. In a small bowl, add oil, lemon juice, and lemon zest and combine. Set aside.

5. Drain the split peas and add them to the large bowl.

6. Drain the bulgur wheat and ensure all water is well-drained before adding this to the bowl with the split peas and vegetables. Mix thoroughly.

7. Add the oil and lemon sauce to the bowl and stir well. Season with salt and pepper to taste and leave to sit for approx. 30 minutes to allow the flavours to develop.

8. Stir in the pomegranates and the sumac and serve.

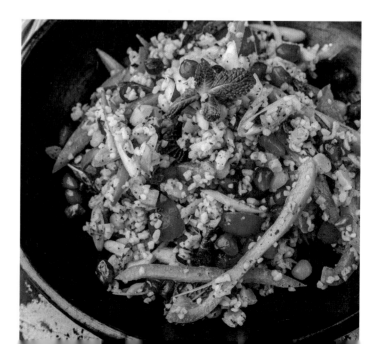

Seabass With Black Rice & Mango Salsa

Serves: 1 | **Difficulty:** Easy | **Total time:** 20 min.

1. Cook the rice as per package instructions.

2. Meanwhile, season the fish with sea salt and black pepper, to taste.

3. Put a non-stick skillet or griddle pan on medium to high heat. Once the pan is hot, drizzle it with olive oil, then fry the fish as per instructions.

4. When ready, serve with fish on a bed of rice, topped with the mango salsa.

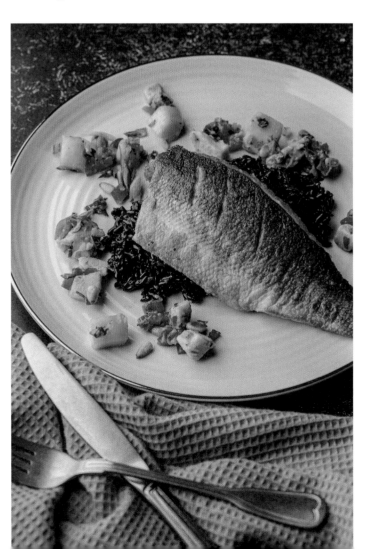

Ingredients

1 filleted white fish (I like halibut or seabass.)

Sea salt and black pepper, to taste

75g uncooked wholegrain rice (or black jasmine rice which is great for a splash of colour)

2 tbsp Mango Salsa (See my recipe in Dips & Spreads.)

1/2 tbsp olive oil

Goat Cheese & Waldorf Salad

Serves: 1 | **Difficulty:** Easy | **Total time:** 30 min.

Ingredients

30g goat cheese

150g Low-fat Greek yoghurt or plain yoghurt

1 tsp Dijon mustard

Juice of 1/2 lemon

80g dark seedless grapes, halved

1 crisp eating apple, halved, cored and thinly sliced

1 stalk of celery, finely sliced

1 handful of lettuce leaves, shredded

30g walnuts, toasted and roughly chopped

Small handful watercress leaves

Sea salt and black pepper to taste

1 tsp sumac

1. Preheat oven to 180°C.

2. Place the goat cheese on a baking tray lined with baking parchment and bake for 20 minutes.

3. Meanwhile, in a bowl, mix together the yoghurt, 1-2 tsp lemon juice, Dijon mustard and combine well.

4. In another large bowl, mix together the grapes, apple, celery and lettuce.

5. Add the yoghurt dressing to the lettuce bowl and mix well. Season as desired with salt and pepper, and extra lemon juice. Stir in the walnuts.

6. Place in a serving bowl, top with watercress, and a sprinkle of sumac and then add the baked goat cheese.

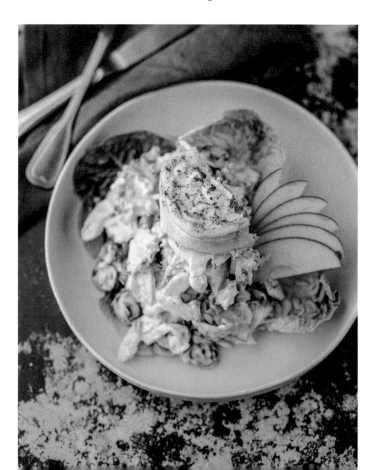

Veggie Tacos

Serves: 2 | **Difficulty:** Easy | **Total time:** 15 min. | Suitable for vegetarians and vegans

1. In a large bowl, add the vegetables, black beans and olive oil. Season with the cumin, paprika, chilli powder, and salt and pepper and mix thoroughly so the vegetables are evenly coated.

2. Heat a large griddle pan on medium to high heat and add the garlic to the pan. Cook for a few minutes until the garlic becomes fragrant.

3. Add all vegetables to the griddle pan and cook for a few more minutes until the vegetables have softened and become slightly charred. Take off the heat and set aside.

4. To crisp up the tortillas, heat a large non-stick frying pan on medium heat. Add the tortillas one at a time, frying for approximately 10 seconds on each side. They should puff up a little and become crispy.

5. To assemble your tacos, add the vegetable mix to the middle of the tortilla, top with salsa, a sprinkle of cheese, jalapenos, and a squeeze of lime juice.

Ingredients

2 tbsp olive oil

1/2 red pepper, diced

1/2 yellow pepper, diced

1/2 green pepper, diced

1 red onion, peeled and cut into thin slices

6 mushrooms, thinly sliced

3 baby corns

6 cherry tomatoes, quartered

100g black beans, drained and rinsed

1/2 aubergine (eggplant), cubed

1 tsp cumin

1 tsp paprika

1 tsp chilli powder

1 garlic clove, crushed

1-2 chillies, diced

1 lime, cut into wedges

4 small wholemeal tortillas

Serve with salsa of your choice — tomato salsa/guacamole, avocado salsa (See my Dips & Spreads.)

20g grated cheddar cheese (optional)

Salt and pepper, to taste

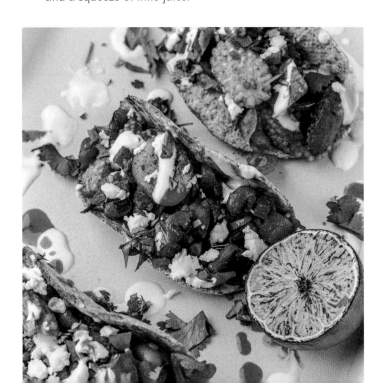

Chicken & Orange Salad

Serves: 2 | **Difficulty:** Easy | **Total time:** 20 min.

Ingredients

2 chicken breasts

1 tbsp olive oil

1 tsp dried smoked paprika

1 orange, zested, peeled and segmented

2 spring onions, slices diagonally

1-2 tsp white wine vinegar

1 tsp clear honey

4 handfuls of mixed salad leaves

1/4 cucumber, halved and finely sliced

6 cherry tomatoes, halved

150g wholegrain rice, cooked as per packet instructions

1 tbsp toasted flaked almonds

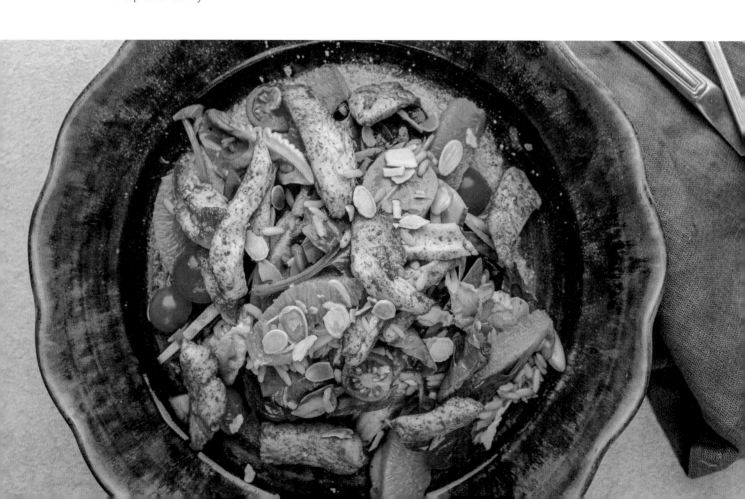

1. Place the chicken breasts between 2 sheets of cling-film and smash with a rolling pin to an even thickness.

2. Coat the chicken with a drizzle of oil and add the smoked paprika.

3. Preheat the grill to medium-high heat.

4. Add the chicken to a griddle pan and place it under the grill, cooking evenly on each side until the chicken is cooked through.

5. Meanwhile, in a small bowl, combine the orange zest, 1 tbsp oil, the white wine vinegar and the honey to make the vinaigrette dressing. Season it as desired with salt and pepper.

6. In a salad bowl, mix together the rice and salad leaves and half of vinaigrette dressing.

7. Place the rice and salad onto serving plates.

8. Top with the orange slices, tomatoes, cucumber slices and spring onions.

9. Slice the chicken and place on top of the salad.

10. Drizzle the remainder of the vinaigrette dressing and top with a sprinkle of flaked almonds.

Sticky Steak Stir Fry

Serves: 1-2 | **Difficulty:** Easy | **Total time:** 20 min.

Ingredients

80g broccoli (I love tenderstem broccoli/broccolini for this recipe!)

1 1/2 tbsp sesame seed oil

65g lean stir fry beef steak strips

1 tsp Chinese 5 Spice

1 garlic clove, crushed

Thumb-size piece of ginger, peeled and grated

4 spring onions, sliced diagonally

60g roasted antipasto peppers in vinegar, drained and sliced

2 baby corn cobs, sliced down the middle

20g carrots, thinly shaved

20g sugar snap peas

1/2 tbsp honey

1/2 tbsp light soy sauce

Juice of 1/2 lime

Small handful fresh coriander leaves

1 red chilli, finely sliced into rounds

1/2 tsp chilli flakes

Salt and black pepper, to taste

Sprinkle sesame seeds

75g uncooked wholegrain rice or wholegrain noodles

1. Add the broccoli to a heatproof bowl and cover in boiling water for a couple of minutes. Drain and refresh with cold water. This cooks the broccoli but keeps the lovely crunch.

2. In a wok or frying pan, heat 1/2 tbsp of the sesame seed oil over medium-high heat, and then fry the steak strips with the Chinese 5 Spice until just done. Remove from the pan and set aside.

3. Begin to cook the rice or noodles as per the package instructions. Heat another 1/2 tbsp of the remaining oil and fry the garlic and ginger for approx. 2 minutes, ensuring the garlic doesn't burn.

4. Add the spring onions, broccoli, antipasto peppers, baby corn cobs, carrots, sugar snap peas and cook for 1-2 minutes.

5. Return the steaks to the pan with the remaining sesame oil if desired, along with the honey, soy sauce and lime juice. Toss together and warm through for another minute or so.

6. Serve on top of a bed of rice or noodles, sprinkle with the fresh coriander, fresh chilli, chilli flakes and sesame seeds and a squeeze of any extra lime juice, as desired.

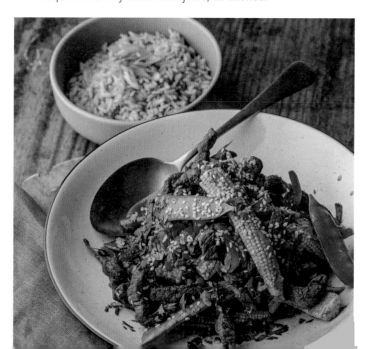

Spaghetti With Tuna, Olives & Capers

Serves: 1 | **Difficulty:** Easy | **Total time:** 20 min.

1. Cook spaghetti as per package instructions.

2. Meanwhile, in a deep frying pan, add 1/2 tbsp oil and garlic over medium-high heat. As soon as the garlic starts to sizzle, add the chilli and fry for 1 minute.

3. Add the tomatoes and fry for another minute.

4. Add 1/2 lemon zest and all the lemon juice, along with salt and pepper to taste, and cook a minute more. Remove from the heat.

5. Drain the spaghetti and add it to the frying pan with the tomatoes.

6. Stir in the tuna, olives and the remaining olive oil. Add in a handful of rocket leaves and gently stir it all together so it's well combined.

7. Serve it up and add a sprinkle of fresh parsley and any extra seasoning or lemon juice as desired.

Ingredients

75g uncooked wholegrain spaghetti

1 tbsp extra virgin olive oil

1 garlic clove, crushed

1/2 medium red chilli, seeded and finely chopped

6 cherry tomatoes, halved

Zest and juice of 1/4 - 1/2 lemon

Handful of rocket leaves

1/2 tsp chilli flakes (if desired)

10g black olives, pitted and roughly chopped

100g tinned tuna, in water, drained and flaked with a fork

Sea salt and black pepper, to taste

Small bunch of fresh parsley, finely chopped

Quick & Easy Homemade Pizza Base

Serves: 1 | **Difficulty:** Easy | **Total time:** 20 min. | Suitable for vegetarians and vegans

Ingredients

1 wholemeal wrap

1 garlic clove, cut in half

Oil spray

100ml tomato passata/strained tomatoes

1/2 tsp mixed herbs

1/2 tsp chilli flakes (optional)

Pizza toppings of your choice – cook as per package instructions.

1. Preheat oven to 240°C.

2. Spray a large baking tray with the oil spray and put the tortilla wrap on it.

3. Spray the top side of the tortilla wrap with oil, then rub the cut side of the garlic all over this side of the wrap.

4. In a small bowl, mix together the tomato passata with the mixed herbs and chilli flakes if desired, and season to taste with salt and pepper.

5. Spread the tomato passata evenly over the top of the wrap, leave a little edge around the tortilla.

6. Depending on the choice of toppings, cook any additional ingredients that need cooking as per package instructions. (The oven is just being used to bake the pizza base and warm the topping ingredients).

7. Top the wrap with the pizza toppings preferred. Add any extra seasonings as desired.

8. Bake in the oven for 4-6 minutes until the wrap is golden brown around the edges, always keeping an eye on it while it is in the oven as the wrap can burn easily.

Healthy Snacks

Always having healthy snacks with you whenever you're out and about, or even when you're at home, can really help you stay on track with eating healthily. If you feel hungry in between meals, having a healthy snack can keep you going and can help prevent your over-eating when you eat your next meal.

For my level of activity, and to help reach my protein goals every day, I regularly include snacks between meals to help meet my nutritional needs. As mentioned previously, protein is really satisfying and can keep you feeling fuller for longer, so I love basing my snacks around this amazing nutrient. In this chapter, I share a bunch of my favourite snacks that I love to make regularly, either for taking to work or for that after dinner snack to satisfy my sweet cravings. Many of these recipes not only provide a source of protein, but a lot of them also contain a great source of fibre or complex carbs to provide you with lots of energy and an extra nutritional boost!

PROTEIN BITES

These little bites of deliciousness are great for getting rid of those hunger pangs that can often creep up on us mid-afternoon, or any time of day for that matter! They're packed full of protein, great for boosting the growth and repair of muscle tissues, and are also a great source of fibre, vitamins and minerals. I love making a batch of these at the weekend to take to work during the week. (See page 229.)

DARK CHOCOLATE BLISS BALLS

If you're like me and have a bit of a sweet tooth, then these hit the spot. They're so addictive and are a great, nutritious way of helping to take away any sugar cravings. They can last in the fridge for a few days, but I also love to put some into an airtight container and store them in the freezer, where they can be kept well for up to three months! (See page 230.)

SPICY CHICKPEAS

These little chickpeas are addictive and great for nibbling on between meals. They are full of flavour and have a delicious crunch. I often make these to take as a snack or to add them in salads or even in my Breakfast Burrito. They're a great source of plant-based protein and fibre. (See page 231.)

PEANUT BUTTER & CRANBERRY ENERGY BALLS

These nutrient powerhouses are packed full of protein, fibre and healthy fats. The sweet and savoury flavours in this recipe make for a delicious combination, and these little bites are honestly so yummy! I love packing a few in my lunch box to go with an afternoon cuppa if I'm in the office. (See page 232.)

PEANUT BUTTER-STUFFED DATES

Dates and peanut butter. Usually when I say that, people turn up their noses. Then they thank me later. Honestly, don't knock it before you try it – the two go surprisingly well together and satisfy your sweet and savoury taste buds. Some self-control is needed with these stuffed dates, though – they're seriously addictive, but just a couple of them make an appropriate serving. (See page 232.)

SALTED CARAMEL BLISS BALLS

Salted caramel is an "in" food these days. I absolutely love it! These energy bites taste just like a sweet and can knock any sugar cravings on the head. They're great for a healthy snack on the go to help boost energy levels, and they take hardly any time to make. (See page 233.)

CHOCOLATE & PEANUT BUTTER BANANA BITES

Have you noticed that I love peanut butter? I really enjoy pairing it with fruit, because it makes such a delicious combination of sweet and savoury flavours, and I find that mixing the two makes for a super-filling snack. These wee bites are so quick and simple to make, they provide a slow release of energy, are packed full of protein, and are great for adding to your lunch bag. (See page 233.)

GREEK YOGHURT WITH FRUIT & NUTS

This is another snack that I regularly have either mid-afternoon or even for supper. I also love having this snack for breakfast sometimes, too. I use Greek yoghurt a lot in my recipes, because it has a really high protein content (about 8g per 100g) which makes it super filling and great for encouraging the growth and repair of muscle tissue. A lot of Greek yoghurts also contain live bacteria, too, as a source of probiotics, which can help to support our gut health. I know many people sometimes find the texture too thick, but a useful tip I always give is to spoon the yoghurt into a bowl then mix it up with a fork first before eating it. This really smooths it out and can make it much nicer to eat. I used to not be very keen on the texture when I first tried it but now I absolutely love it! Greek yoghurt is also naturally low in sugar, but if you feel you need to add a little sweetness, try adding a little honey, maple syrup or vanilla essence. (See page 234.)

MANGO & RASPBERRY CHIA PUDDING

This snack tastes like dessert, too! This pudding is packed full of plant-based protein, Omega-3 fats and vitamins! It's deliciously sweet, and something I often love to have as a snack in the evening, after dinner. (See page 235.)

DEVILLED EGGS – BUFFALO STYLE

I love making boiled eggs for a high protein snack to have on the go but do admit that on their own they can be a little boring. This recipe takes a little extra time to make, but if these flavours work for you, then I guarantee you it's worth the extra effort! (See page 236.)

SPICED OATMEAL, ORANGE & SULTANA COOKIES

This recipe was actually inspired and created for my lovely dad. There's nothing he loves more than a nice cup of tea and a buttery, sultana cookie (or two!). This healthier version got my dad's seal of approval and they are a great option if you need a mid-afternoon pick-me-up, or you have friends popping over for a catch-up. (See page 237.)

APRICOT & CRANBERRY GRANOLA SLICES

This nutrient-packed snack is a great source of carbohydrates and protein to boost energy levels and keep you feeling satisfied. It's full of healthy fats and fibre, and they are super simple and easy to make. If I can't organise a meal immediately after a workout, I love having these as a post-workout snack instead, along with a glass of milk for that extra protein. They keep great for a few days in an airtight container and can even be keep for a couple of months in the freezer, too, so you can take them out whenever you need them. (See page 238.)

DARK CHOCOLATE & CHERRY TRAIL MIX

This recipe is for a great snack to take on the go. I love packing a wee container of this trail mix into my pocket to keep me going at work when I'm running in between wards in the hospital. It's packed full of protein and fibre, and the dried fruit and chocolate add a delicious sweet and rich flavour. That being said, you can really be creative with this recipe on your own, using any nuts and seeds you like. A little reminder that a portion size is roughly about 30g – which is a small handful. (See page 239.)

BANANA & BLUEBERRY MUFFINS

These are a real game changer and a recipe which so many people have asked for. I've shared it before quite a number of times on my social media accounts, and I always get so many people saying how much they like them. The wholemeal flour boosts the fibre content and gives a great texture to the muffins, and the Greek yoghurt provides a great source of protein. I often make these to use up overripe bananas and even have them as a light pre-workout snack on the way to the gym in the morning! (See page 240.)

PICK 'N' MIX RICE CAKES

I love rice cakes and find them a really filling snack to have on the go or for lunch with the right topping! I know many people say they taste bland but with a delicious topping, they can be really tasty and satisfying and a lighter alternative to bread and oatcakes! Here are some of my favourite toppings – a whole mix of savoury and sweet options for you to try out. Be creative and try out your own ideas! (See page 242.)

Protein Bites

Serves: 12 | **Difficulty:** Easy | **Total time:** 30 min.

1. Preheat oven to 200°C.

2. Grease a 12-muffin tray lightly with butter.

3. Mix zucchini, onion, tomatoes, eggs, wholegrain mustard, cheese and chives in a bowl. Season as desired.

4. Place 2 tbsp of the mixture into each cup of the muffin tin.

5. Top with extra grated cheese, a sprinkle of pumpkin seeds, and black pepper.

6. Bake in the oven for 20 minutes.

7. Leave to cool slightly for a few minutes, then remove the muffins from the muffin tray and leave to cool on a wire rack.

Ingredients

1 courgette/zucchini (grated)

1/2 large onion, finely diced

8 cherry tomatoes, finely chopped

5 eggs, beaten

1-2 tsp wholegrain mustard

3 handfuls grated mature cheddar, plus extra for topping

1 tbsp chives, finely chopped

1 tbsp pumpkin seeds

Salt and pepper, to taste

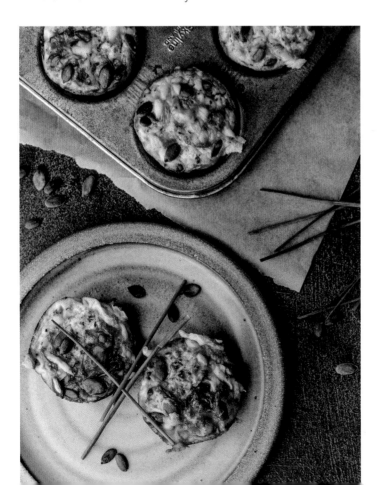

Dark Chocolate Bliss Balls

Serves: 10-12 | **Difficulty:** Easy | **Total time:** 15 min. | Suitable for vegetarians

Ingredients

130g cashew nuts

2 tbsp honey

1 tsp vanilla extract

15 pitted dates

2 tbsp cacao powder

2 tbsp dried coconut or chopped hazelnuts or pistachios (optional)

1. In a food processer, add the cashew nuts and pulse blend to a crumb-like consistency.

2. Then add the honey, vanilla extract, dates and cacao powder and blend it altogether. The mixture should start sticking together. If not, add some extra honey or water. Taste the mixture and adjust the sweetness with extra honey/vanilla extract if required.

3. Roll the mixture into approximately 12 balls, close to the size of a golf ball, and then coat them in the preferred choice of coating, e.g. coconut/hazelnuts/pistachios.

4. To set, place in the fridge on a baking tray for at least 1-2 hours and then store in an airtight container in the fridge.

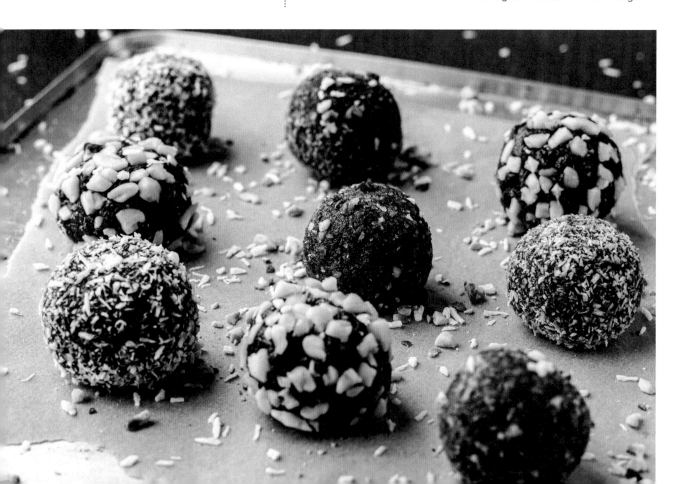

Spicy Chickpeas

Serves: 1 | **Difficulty:** Easy | **Total time:** 40 min. | Suitable for vegetarians and vegans

1. Preheat oven to 180°C.

2. Line a baking tray with baking parchment.

3. Place the chickpeas on the baking tray, drizzle the olive oil over them, and season with the spices, salt and pepper.

4. Toss well until the chickpeas are evenly coated.

5. Bake for 35 minutes, shaking the tray halfway through so they can dry evenly and have become crunchy.

6. Leave to cool, then store in an airtight container.

Ingredients

4 tbsp chickpeas, drained and rinsed

1/2 - 1 tbsp olive oil

1/2 tsp dried paprika

1/2 tsp cayenne pepper

1/2 tsp cumin

Sea salt and black pepper, to taste

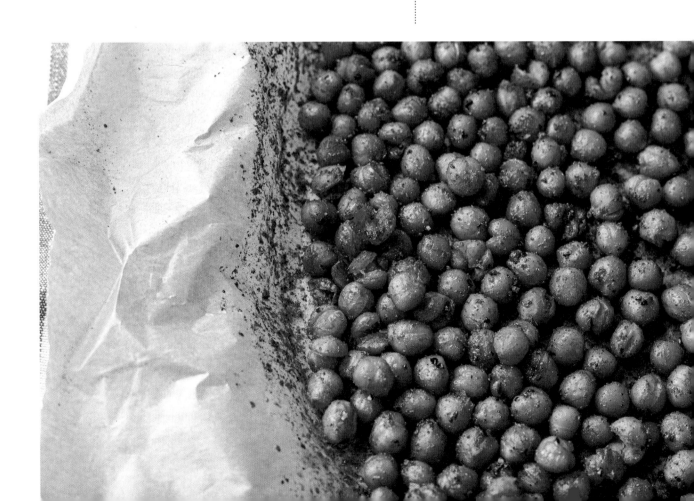

Peanut Butter & Cranberry Energy Balls

Serves: 12 | **Difficulty:** Easy | **Total time:** 20 min. | Suitable for vegetarians and vegans

Ingredients

100g oats

1 tbsp chia seeds

1 tsp cinnamon

1 tbsp dried cranberries

1 tbsp dark chocolate chips (optional)

1 tbsp coconut oil, melted

1/2 tbsp maple syrup or honey

1 tsp vanilla extract

75g crunchy, (no added sugar) peanut butter

1. In a bowl, add the oats, chia seeds, cinnamon, cranberries and dark chocolate chips (if using) and mix together.

2. In another bowl, combine the coconut oil, maple syrup or honey, vanilla extract and peanut butter.

3. Add the wet ingredients to the dry ingredients and mix together using a wooden spoon. A sticky mixture should form. If the mixture is too dry, add more honey/maple syrup or even a little water. If it is too sticky, add some more oats.

4. Separate the mixture into approx. 12 golf ball-sized balls.

5. Place them on a tray and put in the fridge to set before storing in an airtight container in the fridge.

Peanut Butter-Stuffed Dates

Serves: 12 | **Difficulty:** Easy | **Total time:** 5 min.

Ingredients

12 medjool dates, pitted

6 tsp crunchy peanut butter

Optional toppings: dried coconut, crushed pistachios or crushed hazelnuts

1. Slice the dates lengthways and spoon a small amount of peanut butter into each one.

2. Top with preferred toppings.

Salted Caramel Bliss Balls

Serves: approx. 8-10 balls | **Difficulty:** Easy | **Total time:** 20 min. | Suitable for vegetarians and vegans

1. Line a baking tray with baking parchment.

2. Put the cashew nuts in a food processor and pulse until they become crumbly.

3. Add the dates, vanilla essence, maple syrup and sea salt and blend all the ingredients together until well combined. The mixture should be sticky.

4. Roll the mixture into approx. 8-10 golf ball-sized balls and place on the lined baking tray. Refrigerate for approx. 30 minutes before storing in an airtight container in the fridge.

Ingredients

100g unsalted cashew nuts

12 medjool dates, pitted

1/2 tsp vanilla extract

1/2 tbsp maple syrup

Generous pinch of sea salt

Chocolate & Peanut Butter Banana Bites

Serves: 1 | **Difficulty:** Easy | **Total time:** 10 min. + 30-min. setting time | Suitable for vegetarians and vegans

1. Line a baking tray with baking parchment

2. Place half of the banana slices on the baking parchment and top each with a small amount of peanut butter.

3. Put another banana slice on top of each banana slice to make a sandwich with the peanut butter.

4. Put the dark chocolate in a microwavable bowl and heat in the microwave for approx. 30 seconds, making sure the chocolate doesn't burn or solidify. Continue to microwave it until the chocolate has melted and is runny.

5. Using a teaspoon, drizzle the chocolate over the top of the banana sandwiches and promptly sprinkle with desiccated coconut before putting the tray in the fridge to set for approx. 30 minutes.

Ingredients

1 medium banana, peeled and sliced into 1/2 cm-thick slices

100 dark chocolate chips

1 tbsp crunchy peanut butter

Optional: desiccated coconut

Greek Yoghurt With Fruit & Nuts

Serves: 1 | **Difficulty:** Easy | **Total time:** 5 min. | Suitable for vegetarians

Ingredients

100g low-fat Greek yoghurt

1/2 tsp honey (optional)

80g of your choice of fruit – I love mixed berries!

25g toasted flaked almonds

Sprinkle desiccated coconut

1. In a bowl, combine the yoghurt and the honey if used.

2. Top with a preferred choice of fruit, followed by the flaked almonds and coconut.

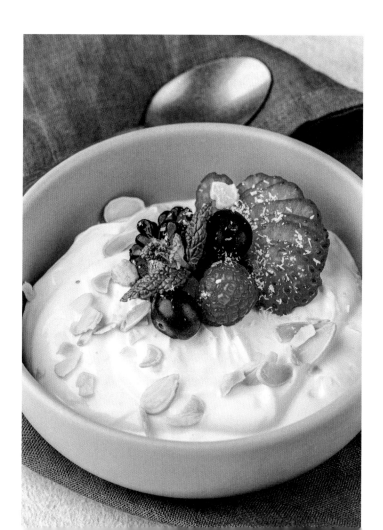

Mango & Raspberry Chia Pudding

Serves: 1 | **Difficulty:** Easy | **Prep time:** 10 min. | **Total time:** 1 hr. 10 min. | Suitable for vegetarians and vegans

1. In a bowl, mix the chia seeds, maple syrup, vanilla essence and coconut milk together.

2. Place the bowl in the fridge to set for approx. 45-60 minutes. When set, the chia seeds should form a gel-like consistency.

3. In a separate bowl, mash the mango until smooth (keeping some separate for topping the pudding).

4. In a third bowl, mash the raspberries with a fork until a thin sauce is formed. To help, heat the raspberries for approx. 15 seconds in the microwave, if needed.

5. In the bottom of a jar or glass, add a layer of the mango, followed by a layer of chia seeds, then all the raspberries. Add a layer of chia seeds and a final layer of mango. Top the pudding with the leftover diced mango and add a sprinkle of desiccated coconut to garnish.

Ingredients

30g chia seeds

1 tbsp maple syrup

1 tsp vanilla extract

200ml unsweetened coconut milk

40g mango, diced

40g raspberries

Sprinkle of desiccated coconut

Devilled Eggs – Buffalo Style

Serves: 1 | **Difficulty:** Easy | **Total time:** 25 min. + 30 min. setting time

Ingredients

2 free-range eggs

Sprinkle of dried paprika, to taste

1/2 tbsp lemon juice

Salt and pepper to taste

10g crumbled blue cheese

1/2 tbsp Buffalo Hot Sauce plus a small amount to drizzle (optional)

1/2 tbsp Dijon mustard

1 tbsp Greek yoghurt

1. In a small-medium saucepan, place the eggs and cover with a few inches of cold water. Bring the water to a boil, then reduce to a slow simmer for approx. 9-10 minutes.

2. Remove the pan from the heat, pour out the hot water and cover the eggs with cold water, and let sit for about 10 minutes until the eggs have cooled enough to allow the shells to be peeled off.

3. Cut the eggs in half lengthways, carefully scoop out the yolk, and put the yolks in a bowl, laying the egg whites on a flat dish.

4. Mash the egg yolks with a fork, then add the Dijon mustard, Greek yoghurt, lemon juice, blue cheese, buffalo sauce and seasoning.

5. Spoon the mixture evenly into the egg whites and store in the fridge for approx. 30 minutes to allow A sprinkle of some extra cheese, buffalo sauce, and paprika gives them a delicious finish!

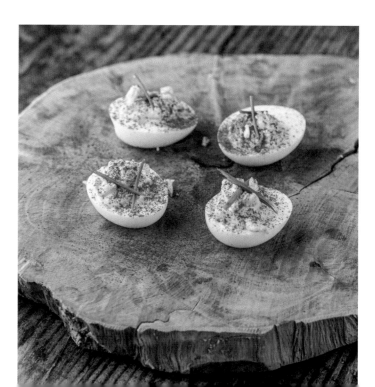

Spiced Oatmeal, Orange & Sultana Cookies

Serves: approx. 8 | **Difficulty:** Easy | **Total time:** 40 min.

1. Preheat oven to 180°C.

2. Line 2 flat baking trays with baking parchment.

3. In a large bowl, combine the oats, flour, baking powder, cinnamon, sultanas and salt.

4. In another bowl, add the butter and honey and beat together until well combined. Add the vanilla extract and the egg, beating them together until well blended. Mix in the orange zest.

5. Gradually add the dry ingredients to the wet ingredients and mix well with a wooden spoon until a thick dough is formed.

6. Put the bowl in the fridge for approx. 10-15 minutes to allow the mixture to stiffen.

7. Using a large spoon, scoop out approx. 10-12 portions of the dough onto the baking trays, allowing for approx. 2 inches of space between each one. Flatten slightly to form even round shapes.

8. Bake in the oven for approx. 15 minutes until golden brown. Optional – sprinkle some light brown sugar over the top of the cookies while they're still hot and just out the oven.

9. Leave the cookies on the baking tray for approx. 5-10 minutes until they set, and then transfer them to a wire rack to finish cooling.

Ingredients

100g instant porridge oats

100g self-rising wholemeal flour, sifted

1 tsp baking powder

3 tsp cinnamon

50g sultanas

100g butter (softened)

Pinch salt

120ml honey

1 free range egg, beaten

1 tsp vanilla extract

1/2 orange, zested

Optional: sprinkle of light brown sugar

Apricot & Cranberry Granola Slices

Serves: approx. 12-14 | **Difficulty:** Easy | **Total time:** 30 min. | Suitable for vegetarians

Ingredients

20g sunflower seeds

20g pumpkin seeds

150g rolled oats

2 tbsp dried coconut

15g flaxseeds

20g dried apricots, cut into small chunks

20g dried cranberries

30g toasted, flaked almonds

4 tbsp peanut butter (I prefer smooth peanut butter for this recipe!)

4 tbsp honey

3 tbsp coconut oil

1. Preheat oven to 180°C.

2. Line a rectangular or square baking tray with baking parchment.

3. In a large mixing bowl, combine sunflower seeds, pumpkin seeds, oats, dried coconut, flaxseeds, apricots, cranberries and toasted, flaked almonds.

4. In a saucepan over low heat, add the peanut butter, honey and coconut oil and stir constantly until all is melted and well blended.

5. Gradually add the ingredients from the saucepan into the bowl with the dry ingredients and stir through with a wooden spoon until all the mixture is well combined. It should be moist and sticky.

6. Spoon the mixture onto the baking tray, spreading it out over the whole tray and pressing the mixture down so it is evenly spread. At this stage, I suggest slightly scoring the top of the granola mixture into the size and shapes preferred – the recipe should make around 12-14 even slices.

7. Bake in the oven for approx. 15 minutes until golden brown. It should be firm to the touch.

8. Remove the granola slab carefully from the baking tray, placing it on either a flat chopping board or wire rack and allow to cool completely before cutting.

Dark Chocolate & Cherry Trail Mix

Serves: 8-10 | **Difficulty:** Easy | **Total time:** 5 min. | Suitable for vegetarians and vegans (if using vegan chocolate)

1. In a large bowl, mix all the ingredients together.
2. Divide the mixture into approx. 8-10 portions and store in an airtight container.

Ingredients

20g sunflower seeds

20g pumpkin seeds

20g dark chocolate chips

20g dried cherries, finely chopped

20g dried cranberries

20g walnuts

15 Brazil nuts, roughly chopped

30g almonds

30g unsalted cashew nuts

30g unsalted peanuts

20g dried coconut flakes

Optional: pinch of salt

Banana & Blueberry Muffins

Serves: 12 | **Difficulty:** Easy | **Total time:** 40 min.

Ingredients

300g wholemeal self-rising flour

1 tsp bicarbonate of soda

50g porridge oats

3 ripe medium bananas, mashed until smooth

100g honey

280ml Greek yoghurt

4 tbsp light olive oil

1 tsp vanilla essence

2 egg whites

140g blueberries

1/2 tbsp light brown sugar for topping (optional)

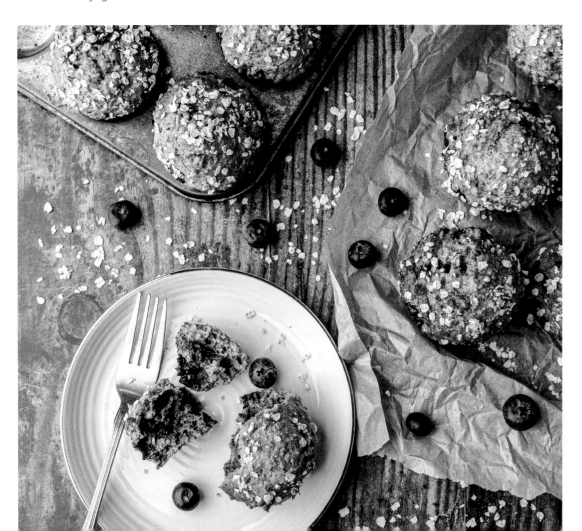

1. Preheat oven to 180°C.

2. Line a 12-muffin tin with paper muffin cups or lightly butter the muffin tin.

3. In a large mixing bowl, sift in the flour and bicarbonate of soda. Add the oats and mix well.

4. In a separate large bowl, add the banana, honey, yoghurt, oil, vanilla essence and egg whites.

5. Add the wet ingredients to the dry ingredients and mix through with a wooden spoon so they're well blended.

6. Gently add the blueberries and stir once or twice until they spread through the mixture to make sure the blueberries don't burst.

7. Divide the mixture evenly into the muffin tin and level out the tops gently with the back of a spoon.

8. Sprinkle the top of the muffins with some extra porridge oats and the light brown sugar if desired.

9. Bake in the oven for approx. 20-25 minutes. The muffins should be well risen, and the tops should be a nice golden brown. To test whether the centre of the muffins are baked, pierce one with a sharp knife. If the knife comes out clean, the muffins are ready.

10. Leave to cool for 10 minutes in the tray then remove them and allow them to finishing cooling on a wire rack.

Pick 'n' Mix Rice Cakes

Serves: 2-3 rice cakes | **Difficulty:** Easy | **Total time:** Quick but variable prep times depending on chosen toppings

Ingredients

Unsalted/plain rice cakes

» *Toppings*

Dark chocolate (melted)

Peanut butter

PLUS fresh or dried fruit

Chia Seed Jam (See my Dips & Spreads.)

Smoked salmon, cream cheese and chive

Pesto

Hummus

Pear, spinach and blue cheese

Avocado and tomato salsa

Cottage cheese

Banana and peanut butter

Tomatoes and sea salt and black pepper

Tuna and cucumber

Boiled egg and hot sauce

Greek yoghurt and honey and fruit

Feta cheese, sundried tomatoes and basil

1. Top rice cakes with one or more of these toppings.

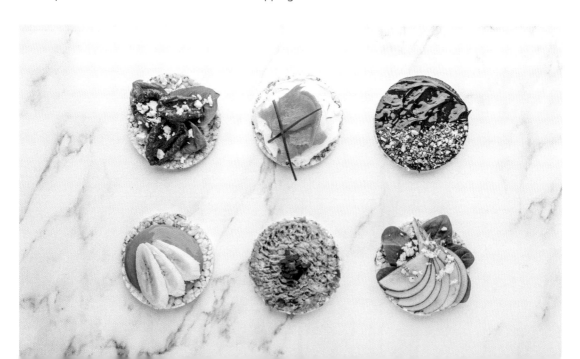

Sweet Indulgence

I've mentioned before that I have a sweet tooth, and there's really nothing that I love more than sitting down and indulging in a cuppa and a piece of cake! I absolutely love delicious, sweet baked goods – I mean everything – cakes, biscuits, pancakes, scones, brownies, you name it – I love it all. And I have my mum and gran to blame (thank) for this. Both of them baked regularly when I was growing up, and I loved helping them out. My mum always has a supply of amazing baked goods ready for any surprise visitors that might pop by, and some of my favourite memories with my lovely gran are of her and me baking up a storm and then devouring what we've made with a warm cup of tea afterwards. This is where my own love for baking started. Baking is now something I do as a hobby and to relax. I love looking for recipe inspiration and then getting in the kitchen and creating something delicious.

I've mentioned a few times throughout the book that I am a Dietitian who truly believes in a balanced diet, and I also believe that every good Dietitian will agree. Contrary to popular belief, Dietitians aren't the 'Food Police', and many of us have actually gone into the profession because of our sheer love for food and the belief that everyone else should be able to find enjoyment from it as well.

Unnecessary restrictions can often lead to periods of binge eating, and binge eating can often be associated with feelings of anxiety, shame and guilt, which can result in the development of a toxic relationship with food. It doesn't need to be that way. Every food has its place in our diet, whether it be for optimising our health or for nourishing our souls. Food is something that I believe should always be enjoyed, especially in company. If whatever diet you are following is making you unhappy, or stops you from enjoying special moments with family and friends, then you need to think about why exactly you're following that diet, what you're gaining from it, and at what expense.

There really is a way to have your cake and eat it, too – it's just about being mindful of how often you eat it and that's why I really believe in the power of nutritional education. By improving your nutritional knowledge, you'll actually want to eat better because you know that it's good for your health. Having this attitude can then allow you the flexibility and freedom to enjoy the more indulgent things in life every now and then, with no feelings of guilt.

The recipes in this section are a few of my sweet favourites that I love to make. They're completely indulgent because I'm not a believer in the 'raw', low-calorie version of things like this. If I'm having a cake, I want the real deal. I hope you enjoy them just as much as I do.

COCONUT, RASPBERRY & WHITE CHOCOLATE MUFFINS

These are little bites of heaven. I love making these for family and friends, and they always go down great. Can you really go wrong with something that has white chocolate in it? AND coconut? (See page 246.)

BERRY BURST BARS

Packed full of nuts and seeds, these sweet and delicious bars provide a load of fibre and a tasty crunch! They take minimal baking skills and there's minimal washing up, too. What's not to love? (See page 247.)

LEMON & VANILLA SHORTBREAD

Anyone who knows me knows just how much I love a good ol' piece of Scottish shortbread. I'm often accused of being 'old' myself for enjoying it so much, but there's really no denying that these crumbly, buttery biscuits are totally delicious. I've put my own twist on the traditional version and added some lemon and vanilla to my recipe. Put the kettle on and just sit back while you enjoy these heavenly delights. (See page 248.)

ZESTY LEMON CAKE

This cake is so light and refreshing and is so, so easy to make. It's a great cake to impress your family and friends with if you're not the keenest of bakers! Give it a go and then get some loved ones round for a cuppa. (See page 250.)

COCONUT BALLS

These little bites of deliciousness are so addictive. They're super simple and easy to make – just don't be afraid to get your hands messy! (See page 251.)

HONEY BUNS

These are another favourite of mine. They go great with a cuppa, and the amazing smell they leave in your kitchen is an added bonus. I love making a fresh batch of these beauties when friends pop over for a coffee and a catch-up. (See page 252.)

CARAMEL SHORTCAKE

Shortbread + caramel + chocolate. Enough said. (See page 253.)

GOOEY CARAMEL BROWNIES

Who doesn't love brownies? They go great with a cuppa or even as a delicious dessert with some ice cream. This recipe is super simple, easy to make, and the addition of caramel really adds something special to the recipe. You can thank me later. (see page 254.)

MUM'S CARROT CAKE

I can take zero credit for this one and owe a huge thank you to my lovely mum for letting me share her amazing recipe with the world. Carrot cake has to be one of my favourite cakes of all time, and I've never had a slice anywhere else that beats my mum's recipe. The crushed pineapple put through this cake keeps the sponge cake so moist and adds a delicious subtle flavour, and the sweet and salty taste from the cream-cheese frosting just tops it all off. This recipe is honestly the definition of heaven on earth. Thank you, Mum! (see page 256.)

Coconut, Raspberry & White Chocolate Muffins

Serves: 12 | **Difficulty:** Easy | **Total time:** 30 min.

Ingredients

375g self-rising flour

90g butter

220g caster sugar

310ml buttermilk (or regular milk)

1 free-range egg, beaten

30g dried coconut (plus extra for topping the muffins)

250g baking white chocolate chips

150g fresh raspberries

1. Preheat oven to 180°C.

2. Line a 12-muffin tin with paper muffin cups or butter the tin, if preferred.

3. In a large bowl, add the flour and then the butter. Rub the flour and butter together with your fingertips, ensuring your hands are dry and cool. Continue to do this until the mixture forms the texture of light breadcrumbs.

4. Add the sugar, buttermilk, egg, dried coconut, chocolate chips and raspberries. Mix them all together, being careful not to burst the raspberries.

5. Divide the mixture between the 12 muffin cups and sprinkle the top with extra dried coconut.

6. Bake the muffins in the oven for approx. 20 minutes. The muffins should be well risen and dark golden on the top. To test whether the centre is cooked, pierce through the centre of a muffin with a sharp knife. The knife should come out clean.

7. Leave the muffins to cool in the tray for approx. 10 minutes before removing them carefully. Set them aside to cool fully on a wire rack.

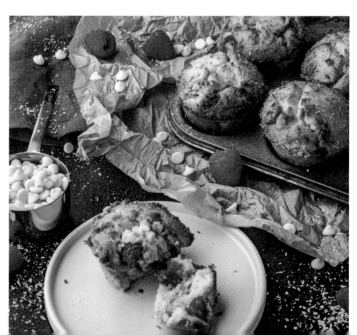

Berry Burst Bars

Serves: 6-8 bars | **Difficulty:** Easy | **Total time:** 25 min.

1. Preheat oven to 200ºC.

2. Line a loaf tin with greaseproof paper.

3. In a small saucepan, melt the butter.

4. Pour the butter into a large bowl and add all the other ingredients. Combine together with a spoon.

5. Pack the mixture into the loaf tin and spread it over the whole tin evenly.

6. Bake in the oven for approx. 30 minutes until the mixture begins to get crispy on top.

7. Leave it to cool for at least 15 minutes before removing it from the tin and cutting it into approx. 6-8 bars.

Ingredients

50g butter

3 tbsp sunflower seeds, roughly chopped

3 tbsp pumpkin seeds, roughly chopped

3 tbsp sesame seeds, roughly chopped

1 ripe banana, mashed

100g oats

30g flaxseeds

50g cranberries

3 tbsp golden syrup

Lemon & Vanilla Shortbread

Serves: approx. 6-8 shortbread triangles | **Difficulty:** Easy | **Total time:** 60 min.

Ingredients

225g plain flour

115g corn flour

115g powdered sugar

225g salted butter, sliced

Pinch of salt

Zest of 1 lemon

1 tsp vanilla essence

1/2 tbsp caster/baker's sugar

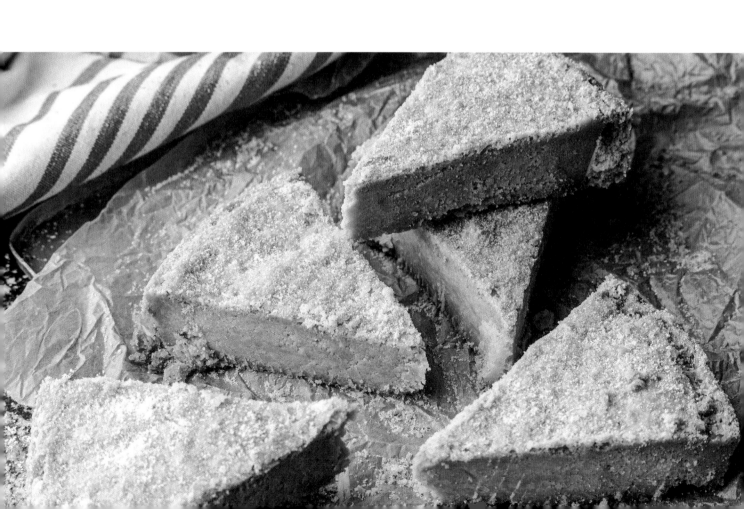

1. Preheat oven to 170°C.

2. In a large bowl, sift the flour, corn flour, powdered sugar, and salt and mix together.

3. Add the butter slices to the flour. Rub in the butter to the flour to form a crumbly texture.

4. Add the lemon zest and vanilla essence and stir them through the flour mixture.

5. Drop the mixture onto a lightly floured surface and knead to form a soft dough.

6. Place the dough on a baking sheet lined with greaseproof paper. Push or roll the mixture out until it's approximately 1cm thick and in your desired shape – which could be square, round, or rectangle. If the dough splits or tears, just press it back together – but remember, the less the dough is worked, the shorter and better these biscuits will be. If you prefer, you can choose to press the dough directly into a greaseproof paper lined baking pan of your choice, to form your desired shape.

7. Score light lines on the shortbread making the shape preferred (e.g. finger slices, triangles, squares etc.). This will allow the shortbread to be cut easier after baking.

8. Put the baking sheet (or baking tin) into the oven and bake for 30-45 minutes. The shortbread should be a lovely light golden colour when it's done.

9. After removing the shortbread from the oven, sprinkle the top with caster/baker's sugar while it's still hot.

10. Leave for 10 minutes if the mixture has been baked in a baking tin, then allow to cool fully on a wire rack before cutting.

Zesty Lemon Cake

Serves: 8-10 | **Difficulty:** Easy | **Total time:** 50 min.

Ingredients

100g softened margarine

175g caster/baker's sugar

175g self-rising flour

1 tsp baking powder

2 large free-range eggs, beaten

4 tbsp milk

Zest and juice of 1 lemon

100g caster/baker's sugar or granulated sugar

1. Preheat oven to 180°C.

2. Lightly grease and line a deep round cake tin with greaseproof paper, (cake size: 7 inches).

3. In a large bowl, combine the softened margarine, caster/baker's sugar, flour, baking powder, eggs, milk and lemon zest. Set approximately 1 tsp lemon zest aside for decorating. Beat all the ingredients in the bowl until smooth and well combined

4. Pour the mixture into the cake tin and level out the surface.

5. Bake in the oven for approximately 35 minutes. The cake should come away slightly from the sides of the baking tin, and the sponge cake should spring back when lightly pressed.

6. Meanwhile, put the lemon juice and 100g caster or granulated sugar in a bowl and stir until well combined.

7. When the cake is ready, remove from the oven and carefully tip the cake tin upside down onto a flat surface to remove the sponge from the tin. Take off the grease proof paper. Carefully turn the sponge back to an upright position and place on a wire rack.

8. Spoon and spread the lemon juice/sugar paste over the top of the sponge while the cake is still hot. Add the remaining lemon zest by sprinkling this over the top of the cake.

9. Leave the sponge to cool and set on the wire rack before serving.

Coconut Balls

Serves: 24 | **Difficulty:** Easy | **Total time:** 15 min. + 1 hr. setting time

1. In a large bowl, combine the coconut, powdered sugar and condensed milk.

2. Using your hands, roll only small amounts of the mixture at a time to form approx. 24 golf ball-sized balls. Place them on a sheet of greaseproof paper on top of a flat plate or tray. If the mixture isn't sticking together, add small amounts of either coconut or powdered sugar and mix well until the right consistency is reached.

3. Melt the chocolate in the microwave or over the stove, whichever is preferred.

4. Dip the balls in the chocolate and make sure they are completely covered.

5. Optional, sprinkle the outside of the balls with more desiccated coconut, if desired.

6. Place the balls back on baking tray.

7. Leave to set in the fridge for at least 1 hour.

Ingredients

250g desiccated coconut

200g powdered sugar

1 tin condensed milk

450g milk chocolate for baking

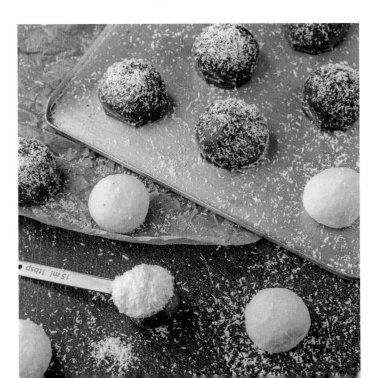

Honey Buns

Serves: 12 | **Difficulty:** Easy | **Total time:** 35 min.

Ingredients

3 heaped tsp mixed spice

1 tsp bicarbonate of soda

115g margarine

225g sugar

225g raisins

340ml water

1 free-range egg, beaten

450g self-rising flour

1. In a large pot, add the mixed spice, bicarbonate of soda, margarine, sugar, raisins and water and bring to a boil. Simmer for approximately 5 minutes.

2. Leave in the pot until the mixture has completely cooled.

3. When the mixture has cooled, add the egg and flour and mix well until thoroughly blended.

4. Line a 12-muffin tray with paper muffin cups and evenly pour the mixture into each one.

5. Bake in the oven for approximately 20 minutes until the buns have risen well and are golden brown. Test the centre by piercing with a sharp knife – the knife should come out clean.

6. Leave the buns to cool for 5-10 minutes in the muffin tray before removing them carefully and placing them to cool fully on a wire rack.

Caramel Shortcake

Serves: approx. 10 large squares | **Difficulty:** Easy | **Total time:** 30 min.

1. Mix the digestive biscuits and melted butter together and press into a square baking tray which has been lined with greaseproof paper.

2. In a medium pan, melt the condensed milk, caster/baker's sugar and butter together and allow to boil for 5 minutes. Stir regularly.

3. Spread the condensed milk mixture over the digestive biscuits.

4. Melt the milk chocolate either in the microwave or in a bowl over a pot of hot water on the stove.

5. Spread the milk chocolate over the condensed milk mixture.

6. Melt the white chocolate and drizzle horizontal lines of it on top of the milk chocolate, leaving about 2cm in between and making sure the lines are evenly spread out. While it's still warm, drag a skewer, toothpick or the tip of a knife through the chocolate to make a feathered pattern on the top.

7. Set aside or place in the fridge until the chocolate has set then carefully remove the shortcake from the baking tin before cutting into squares.

Ingredients

18 digestive biscuits, crushed (Digestive biscuits are a type of semi-sweet biscuit, originating from Scotland. Not from the UK? Try your Imported Food aisle. You may also use graham crackers, but please note texture may affect the result.)

5oz butter

385g condensed milk

6oz caster/baker's sugar

5oz butter

200g bar of milk chocolate

50g white chocolate for baking

Gooey Caramel Brownies

Serves: 12 | **Difficulty:** Easy | **Total time:** 50 min.

Ingredients

200g salted butter

150g milk chocolate, as preferred

50g baking white chocolate

400g tinned caramel

200g golden caster/baker's sugar

4 free range eggs, beaten

1 tsp vanilla essence

130g plain flour

Pinch of salt

2 tbsp cocoa powder

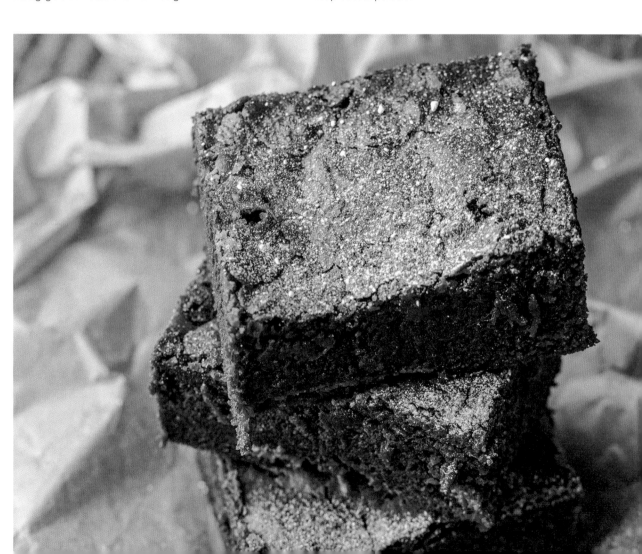

1. Preheat oven to 180°C.

2. Grease and line a deep rectangular baking tin.

3. In a medium saucepan, melt the butter then remove it from the heat.

4. Add the milk chocolate and white chocolate to the butter and stir continuously until all the chocolate has melted.

5. Put 100g of the tinned caramel in a small bowl, mix with a fork to soften and set aside.

6. Add the remaining caramel to a large bowl, along with the golden caster/baker's sugar, eggs and vanilla essence, and beat together with a whisk.

7. Add the butter and chocolate mix in the saucepan to this large bowl and whisk together.

8. Sift the flour, cocoa powder and a pinch of table salt into the mixture and beat well with a wooden spoon until smooth.

9. Transfer the mixture to the baking tin and smooth the surface until it is evenly spread.

10. Taking a teaspoon of the caramel at a time, make around 6-8 stripes of caramel horizontally across the batter.

11. Run a skewer, toothpick or sharp knife vertically through the stripes to make a feathered appearance.

12. Place the tin in the oven and bake for approximately 40 minutes, until the batter is well risen and the top is evenly coloured, forming a firm crust.

13. Leave to cool in the tin, then transfer the brownies to a cutting board. Cut into approximately 12 squares.

Mum's Carrot Cake

Serves: approx. 10 | **Difficulty:** Moderate | **Total time:** 1 hr., 45 min.

Ingredients

» *Sponge*

1 cup oil

11oz sugar

12oz plain flour

1 tsp cinnamon

2 tsp bicarbonate of soda

1 tsp salt

1 small tin crushed pineapple plus juice

8oz carrot, grated

5oz desiccated coconut

3 large eggs

» *Cream cheese icing*

4oz full fat cream cheese

1 tbsp milk

1/4 tsp vanilla essence

1 tsp salt

11oz icing sugar

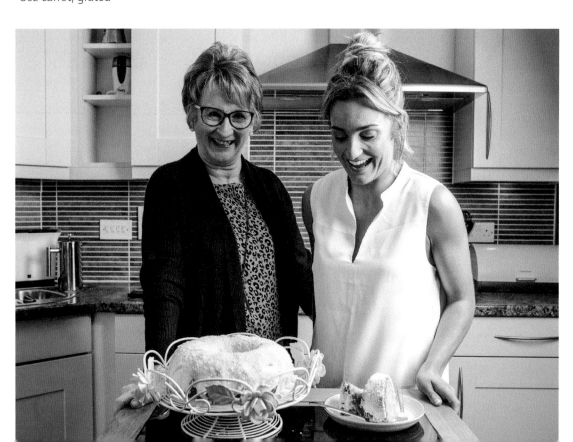

1. Preheat oven to 170°C.

2. Grease and flour a large Bundt baking tin.

3. In a large bowl, beat the eggs, oil and sugar together.

4. In a separate bowl, combine flour, cinnamon, baking soda and salt.

5. In another bowl, combine pineapple, carrot and coconut.

6. Add the pineapple mixture to the egg mixture and stir well.

7. Add the flour mixture to the egg and pineapple mixture and blend together.

8. Pour the cake batter into the Bundt tin.

9. Place in the oven and bake for 1 hour and 15 minutes.

10. Meanwhile, blend the cream cheese, milk, vanilla essence and salt in a large bowl.

11. Gradually add the icing sugar, mixing well until the icing is of spreading consistency. Place the icing in the refrigerator to harden.

12. Once the cake has cooled, spread on the cream cheese icing and sprinkle with the extra desiccated coconut.

Dips & Spreads

Making your own healthy dips and spreads at home can be a great way of using up some leftover ingredients in your kitchen and can really add a delicious hit to some of your favourite dishes. Not only that, but they're great for dipping in some of your favourite veggie sticks or crackers to make a healthy snack, or as a movie night treat with some tortilla chips!

MANGO SALSA

This is also a favourite of mine. Super simple, easy to make and really refreshing, it goes great with fish and as a side dish to curries. (See page 260.)

SPICY TOMATO SALSA

This fiery little number goes great with my Veggie Tacos and mixed in with my Black Bean Breakfast Burrito. I also love using it as a dressing in wraps, on sandwiches, and it's delicious over nachos. (See page 261.)

BEETROOT HUMMUS

Just the colour of this dip will tempt you! It's so bright, and the rich purple colour just screams nutrients! This dip is delicious with your favourite veggie sticks or with some flat bread or wholegrain crackers! (See page 261.)

AVOCADO SALSA

I love avocado on its own, but much prefer to spice it up a little bit by adding a little extra flavour to it. I make this one so often to eat with poached eggs and toast and it's also lovely served up as guacamole to go with Mexican-style dishes. (See page 262.)

LEMON & CORIANDER HUMMUS

I love adding this as a spread to sandwiches or using as dip for veggie sticks to make a healthy snack. It's packed full of plant-based protein and is super filling! (See page 263.)

CHIA SEED JAM

Who would have known that making your own jam can be so easy?! I make this all the time to spread over toast or to stir through my porridge or yoghurt! So simple and easy to make, it contains just a few ingredients and is packed full of plant-based protein and omega 3 fats! Store it in an airtight container in the refrigerator, and it can last up to a week! (See page 264.)

Mango Salsa

Serves: 3-4 | **Difficulty:** Easy | **Total time:** 10 min. | Suitable for vegetarians and vegans

Ingredients

2 mangoes, peeled, stoned and cubed

2 avocados, peeled, stoned and roughly chopped

Small bunch fresh coriander, roughly chopped

1/2 red onion, finely chopped

1 fresh red chilli, finely chopped

1 tbsp extra virgin olive oil

Juice and grated zest of 1 lime

1 tbsp apple cider vinegar

3 spring onions, roughly chopped

1/2 red bell pepper, roughly chopped

Sea salt and black pepper, to taste

1 tbsp pine nuts (toasted)

1. Combine all ingredients in a large bowl and serve as desired.

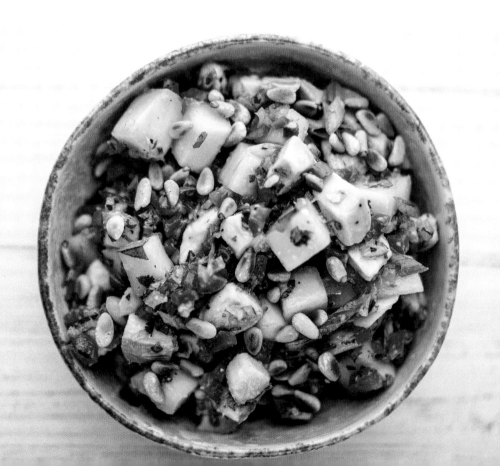

Spicy Tomato Salsa

Serves: 2-3 | **Difficulty:** Easy | **Total time:** 10 min. | Suitable for vegetarians and vegans (if using vegan friendly balsamic vinegar)

1. Combine all ingredients in a large bowl and serve as desired.

Ingredients

Small bunch fresh basil, finely chopped

1/2 fresh red chilli, finely chopped

4-5 sun-dried tomatoes, finely chopped

Juice of 1 lemon

1 tbsp extra virgin olive oil

1/2 tbsp balsamic vinegar

Sea salt and black pepper, to taste

Beetroot Hummus

Serves: 3-4 | **Difficulty:** Easy | **Total time:** 15 min. | Suitable for vegetarians and vegans

1. Blend the chickpeas, the crushed garlic clove and lemon juice in a food processor until smooth.
2. Add the beetroot, yoghurt and olive oil and blend again until a smooth, creamy texture is formed.
3. Season with salt and pepper and extra lemon juice if desired.
4. Place into a bowl and add a drizzle of oil over the top before serving.

Ingredients

240g chickpeas, drained and rinsed

1 garlic clove, crushed

Juice of 1 lemon

250g cooked beetroot, roughly chopped

2 tbsp Greek yoghurt

Salt and pepper, to taste

1 tbsp olive oil (plus extra to drizzle over before serving)

Avocado Salsa

Serves: 2 | **Difficulty:** Easy | **Total time:** 10 min. | Suitable for vegetarians

Ingredients

1 avocado, peeled, stone removed

4 cherry tomatoes, finely chopped

Juice of 1/2 lime

1/2 tsp chilli flakes

Salt and pepper, to taste

1/4 red onion, finely chopped

1. Mash the avocado in a bowl

2. Add the remaining ingredients to the bowl and stir gently to combine.

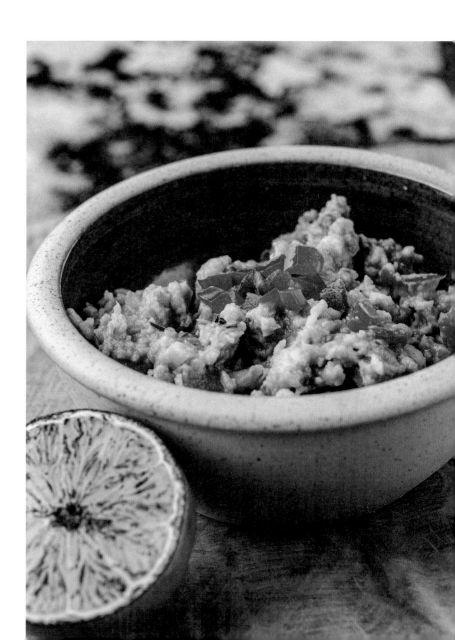

Lemon & Coriander Hummus

Serves: 4-5 | **Difficulty:** Easy | **Total time:** 10 min. | Suitable for vegetarians

1. Add all the ingredients to a food blender/processor, except the coriander. Pulse until smooth.

2. Season to taste.

3. When ready to serve, add a drizzle of olive oil over the top.

Ingredients

400g chickpeas, drained and rinsed

3 cloves garlic

4 tbsp extra virgin olive oil

4 tbsp water

2 tbsp tahini

2 tsp smoked paprika

Salt and black pepper, to taste

Handful of fresh coriander

Juice of 1 lemon

2 tbsp Greek yoghurt

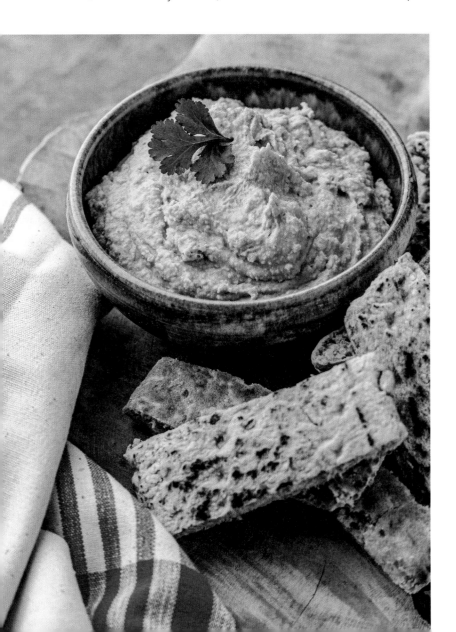

Chia Seed Jam

Serves: 3-4 | **Difficulty:** Easy | **Total time:** 20 min. | Suitable for vegetarians

Ingredients

250g strawberries, tops removed and quartered

200g raspberries

3 tbsp honey

2 tbsp chia seeds

1. Place the strawberries, raspberries and honey in a non-stick pot and heat at a medium setting.

2. Cook for approximately 5 minutes until all the fruit is soft. Stir the fruit continuously, mashing the fruit into a pulp as it becomes softer. The mixture should be quite smooth. Turn the heat down if the mixture starts to boil and all the fruit hasn't been mashed yet.

3. Add the chia seeds and stir thoroughly, leaving on low heat for about 10 minutes. Stir regularly.

4. Put the mixture into a bowl or your desired jar or container to cool. The jam will continue to thicken as it cools.

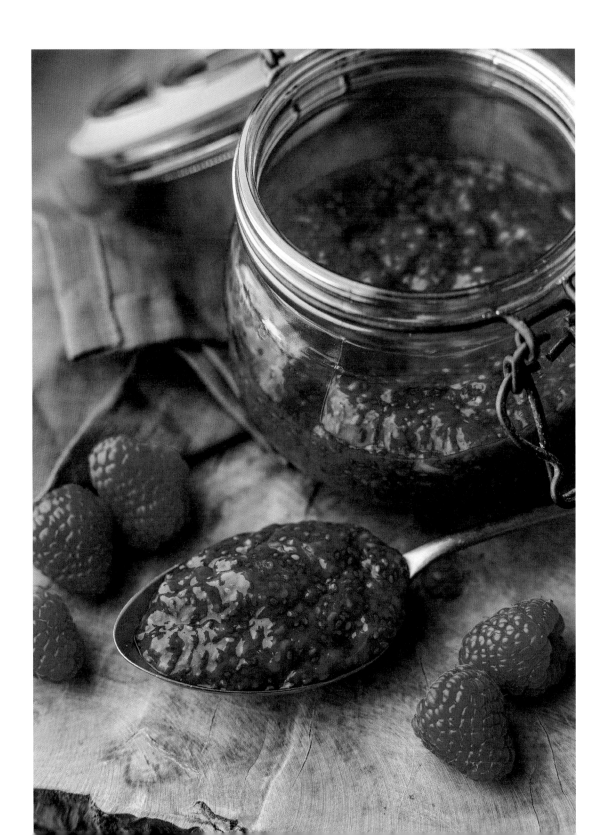

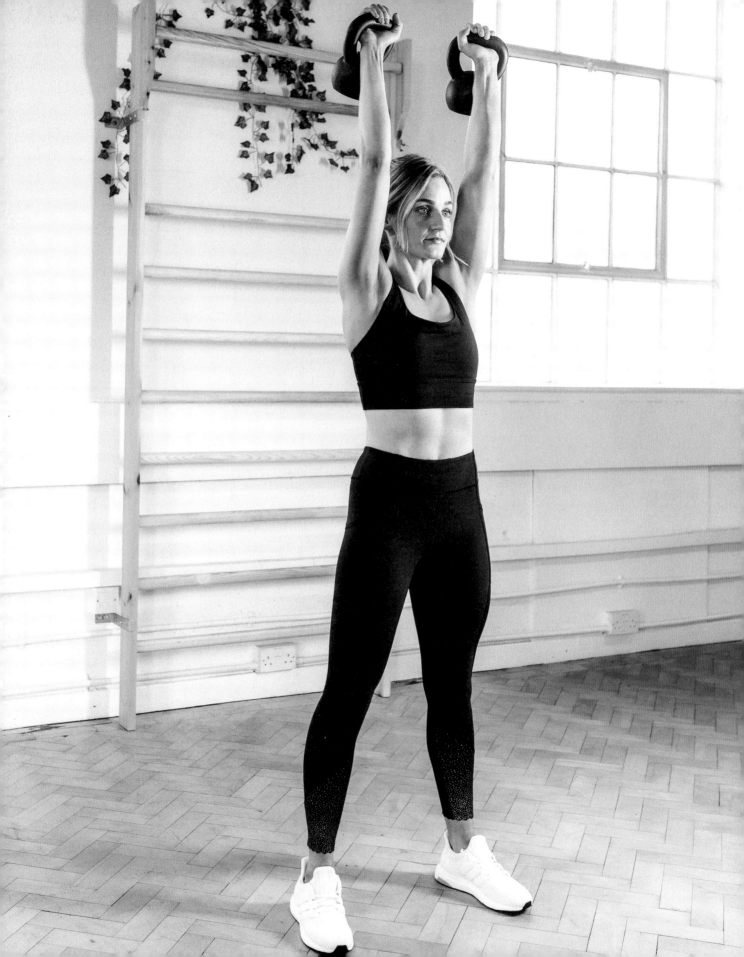

LET'S GET

Active

I've been into sports and exercise from a really young age, and I have my parents to thank for that. They let me try out a number of fun and active kid classes when I was young and encouraged me to try new things at after school clubs when I was in primary school. I loved dancing, netball, horseback-riding and so much more, but my true passion turned out to be athletics. I started doing athletics in primary school where I developed my love for running and was good at a lot of the track and field events, too.

After moving on to high school, I was desperate to keep this up and ended up joining a local athletics club. I loved it. We trained twice a week and had races on Saturdays. Short-distance sprints were always my thing, and I loved the thrill of racing and competing. I kept this up for four years then somewhat regrettably gave it all up once exams became more important at school. I was a conscientious pupil, and I put a lot of pressure on myself to do well at exams that I made the decision to leave the athletics club. Committing so much time to athletics every week was challenging, and I was also trying to juggle having a weekend job and some form of social life, too. I know it was the right decision for me at the time, but I have missed athletics ever since. I have thought about joining an athletics club again a number of times, but now I have developed a passion for so many other types of training, not just athletics.

After giving up athletics halfway through high school, I never made the effort to find any other form of exercise to replace it. There was definitely a short period of time in my life when I did little to no exercise, apart from P.E. at school. I remember going out for a run one day near where my parents live, and for someone who was previously really good at running, I really struggled to run any length of distance before becoming so out of breath that I had to stop. That really hit home with me and gave me the motivation to get back into exercising again. I felt so unfit compared to what I was capable of before.

I started by joining a local gym where I found my love for group fitness. I tried out so many different classes, mainly aerobic and spinning classes, because it was the cardio side of things that I was used to, and I didn't know anything about using weights. I started to run again and quickly saw my running ability improve. I began testing my running out on the treadmills in the gym once I plucked up the courage to get on one of them, and that's when I started noticing how many calories I was burning. I became somewhat obsessed by this, and pairing this up with becoming more and more aware of the calories I was eating at the same time, didn't make for a good combination. I became overly fixated on how many calories I was 'burning', how much I was eating, and how it affected my weight. I weighed myself far too often, and it was only making me miserable. Food and exercise used to be fun, and I had totally lost sight of that.

After starting university and learning more and more about nutrition, it quickly became apparent to me that I was getting it all wrong. I noticed just how inaccurate it was to have a computer on a treadmill telling me how many calories I had burned. I realised that counting calories was only ever going to give me an estimate and I began to understand the importance of focusing on nutrition and exercise for health rather than weight. This is where everything changed for me. My first step was throwing out my bathroom scales. That was one of the best and most rewarding things I have ever done. I started to run outside again, competing only with myself for how fast I could run a certain distance, rather than how far I had to run to burn a certain number of calories.

I joined in some of the strength classes at the gym and found a love for functional circuits and kettlebell classes. My relationship with food and exercise began to improve, and I started to see changes, not only in my body shape, but also in my mood, my skin, my hair – everything. Since then, over the years I've tried out many different types of exercise. My running has always been pretty consistent, but I've gone from doing group fitness classes to following online workout programmes, which I either used to do in the gym or in my garage at home. I had found my love for fitness again and this was really what inspired me to find a way of helping others to do the same.

I began researching what it takes to become a fitness instructor and personal trainer and worked hard to save up the money to join the courses. It was great to learn more about the physiology of the body and how there are so many different ways of training and different training methods that can be used to help reach your goals. With the knowledge I gained from completing these courses, I then started to plan my own training sessions in the gym to see how the training principles worked on me. I did this for ages, but if I'm totally honest, I got bored of my own company. For the most part, I had been so used to exercising with other people. I've always loved the support and motivation that working out with others gives you.

I then decided to try out a local CrossFit gym to see what all the fuss was about. I loved it! I loved the combination of the different types of functional training involved, including cardio, strength, mobility and gymnastics. But the main thing? I absolutely loved exercising with other people again. There's so much encouragement and motivation at every class that it really pushes you to do your best. Two years on and I'm still there but now I mix up my training each week, and I have finally found the right balance for me. In an ideal week, I now run once or twice a week, I do CrossFit a few times a week and I train myself a few times a week by either doing strength sessions or High-Intensity Interval Training (HIIT) sessions. I exercise now for the challenge, for the endorphins, for the fun, for the friendship, for the health benefits, the list goes on. I exercise now for everything but the calories burned.

So I strongly encourage you once again to look for another reason to exercise rather than doing it just to burn calories or to lose weight. If you find a form of exercise you love, it can honestly be one of the most rewarding things ever for so many reasons, and you'll get so much more from exercising than just trying to see how it influences the number on the scales.

I can guarantee you there is some form of exercise out there for everyone, maybe you just haven't found the right one for you yet. Be brave and get out there and try something new – you never know how much you'll love something if you don't give it a try.

By incorporating both cardio and strength training into your routine each week and doing this alongside consuming a healthy and well-balanced diet, you will start to begin your journey towards a healthier, fitter, stronger and happier you. Remember, if you can focus on eating well and exercising for reasons other than weight loss, you are more likely to stay with it and, as a result, your weight will more than likely take care of itself.

To inspire you to get started or to try out something new, I have included a fun series of workouts here for you! In the Getting Active section of the book, we discuss the benefits of both cardiovascular training and strength training and exactly why it's important for you to include both types of exercise in your weekly routine to support and improve your health. I've mentioned lots of times already that you should look for a form of exercise that is suitable for you and that you absolutely love. It doesn't matter what you do or how you do it, as long as you do something that involves these two types of training, then you will reap the benefits.

The type of training that I've provided you with here is a form of anaerobic cardio exercise, which I love doing myself, called High Intensity Interval Training (HIIT). It's a popular form of training because it involves repeated bouts of high intensity exercise with regular and well-timed rest intervals. This allows for a suitable recovery time so that the exercise remains manageable. I love this kind of training because it encourages you to give your maximum effort with the comfort of knowing that you have a recovery period coming up. It can be done by simply using your own body weight or by adding in some weights or resistance bands to make it more challenging!

I am a huge fan of HIIT-style training, and I incorporate it a lot into my own workouts each week. HIIT-style training is also a style of training that is used often in CrossFit workouts. It is short and effective, but challenging. It is a great style of training to use if you are a busy person and you find it difficult to find the time to exercise. Not only that, but you can adapt the workouts very easily to suit your needs. You can do it with or without weight or equipment, you can do it at the gym or at home, you can work your entire body, or you can decide to just focus on the upper or lower body. It's entirely up to you. The short, sharp intervals of high intensity exercise, followed by a rest period, can help to keep you motivated and really encourage you to push yourself. HIIT will not only improve your stamina and endurance, but it will also help you to build muscle, lose fat and improve your cardiovascular health and conditioning. HIIT can also be done in lots of different ways by making use of a variety of HIIT training methods. This keeps your exercising efforts interesting, allowing you to mix up your workout every time!

I have provided you with a series of progressive exercises which are suitable for a Beginner, Intermediate or Advanced level to allow you to choose the workout that's right for you. I have programmed the workouts in such a way so that all major muscle groups will be used, allowing you to do a full-body workout. I have also indicated which exercises work your lower body and those which work your upper body so that you can focus on working just one area in a training session, if you wish.

You will notice that each of the workout levels are programmed in a similar way. The lower body exercises contain 3 basic movement patterns: a squat, a hinge, and a lunge. I have also included a fourth lower body exercise, a hip extension, to help strengthen your glutes. The upper body contains a push and pull exercise, as well as two which will target your core. There may be some exercises that you will progress quicker with than others, so you can also pick and choose different exercises from the other workout levels so you can develop a workout which is suitable for your fitness level.

Additionally, I have indicated which exercises require an essential piece of equipment. The Beginner Level can be done with no equipment, by just simply using your own body weight. For the Intermediate and Advanced Levels, some of the exercises require a few pieces of essential equipment. For the remaining exercises, appropriate equipment has been suggested so that you can increase the intensity of the workout, if you wish. This means that some of the exercises can still be done just by using your own body weight, so you can choose a workout intensity which is right for you.

If you haven't tried a certain exercise before, I always recommend that you practice the movement first, just using your own body weight. This is to ensure that you feel comfortable doing the exercise, and you should master the movement technique before adding in any extra weight or resistance. This can help prevent injury and sometimes using your own body weight is challenging enough. When you feel ready, you can start to gradually add in additional weight to challenge yourself. If you are unsure, please seek help and advice from a qualified exercise professional.

There are seven HIIT training methods you can use to complete your chosen exercises. This allows you to mix up your workout every time, keeping it fun and interesting.

The number of repetitions I recommend in the various training methods is 10 for each exercise. This number of repetitions will encourage muscular hypertrophy, which means building lean muscle mass. The optimal repetition range for muscular hypertrophy is between 6-12 repetitions using a moderate weight. This may just be using your own body weight depending on your fitness level.

If you wish to improve muscular endurance, I recommend completing between 12-20 repetitions of an exercise using a lighter weight. Muscular endurance refers to the ability of a muscle to repeatedly apply force against resistance without becoming tired. So if you wish to improve your muscles' ability to work over a longer period of time, decrease the weight you are using, and do a higher number of repetitions. This higher repetition range can also be appropriate for using in HIIT.

With regards to improving muscular strength, this is best performed with a focus on one or two exercises at a time and is not considered appropriate for HIIT. Muscular strength is the maximum force a muscle (or muscle group) can produce. If you wish to plan your own muscular strength sessions, I would recommend completing between 1-5 repetitions of an exercise using a heavier weight, and doing 2-5 sets, taking 3-5 minutes rest between each set. So if you want to become stronger, aim to gradually increase the weight you use for each exercise, over a number of weeks. Before lifting heavier weights, you must always ensure your exercise technique is correct first to prevent injury.

I generally recommend doing HIIT training two or three times per week, ensuring you spread these sessions out over the week. This will allow time for your body to recover, but will also make sure it doesn't impact on any other training you do (e.g. specific strength sessions or aerobic cardio sessions such as brisk walking, running, swimming etc.).

One more thing before you get started! Make sure you keep track of your workouts – keep a record of the training method used, the weight used and any workout times, to keep track of your progress!

LET'S GET ACTIVE!!

Disclaimer: If you are unsure whether this exercise programme is right for you, always consult your doctor and speak to a qualified exercise professional for more advice.

A few notes before you begin:

Equipment

» I have documented which exercises require an ESSENTIAL piece of equipment for the movement to be carried out.

» Other equipment variations are possible, if preferred. I have demonstrated using my preferred choice of equipment for that particular exercise. If you choose an alternative piece of equipment to that which is demonstrated, make sure you seek advice from a qualified exercise professional on how to use the equipment safely.

Repetitions

» For exercises involving the use of one arm or leg at a time, make sure you complete the recommended number of repetitions on each side.

Warm-Up/Cool-Down

» Ensure you effectively warm up and cool down before and after exercising.

Tracking Progression

» Keep a note of what weights you use for each exercise and your workout times to allow you to track your progress.

» If you feel you are progressing in a certain exercise more than others, you can pick and choose an alternative option from the Beginner, Intermediate or Advanced workout levels to complete the same movement pattern.

THE DIETITIAN KITCHEN HITT WORKOUT

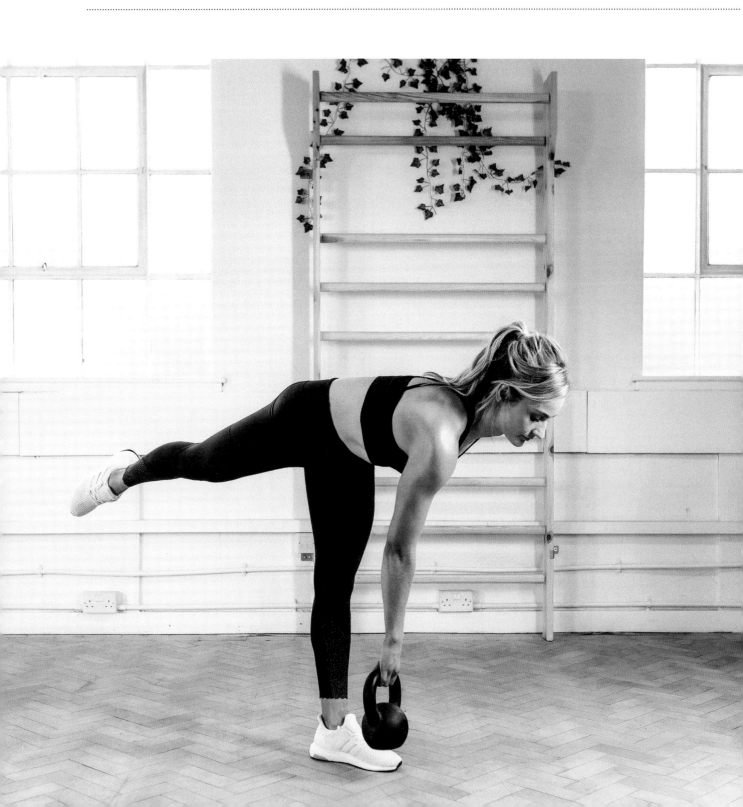

BEGINNER LOWER BODY EXERCISES

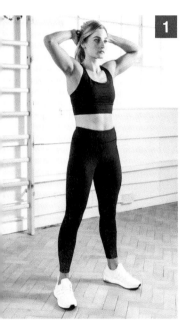

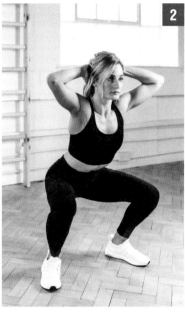

Prisoner Squat

Movement pattern: squat | **Equipment:** none

1. Place both hands behind your head, with one hand on top of the other.

2. Feet should be positioned at shoulder-width apart and toes slightly turned out.

3. Squat down, sending your hips back, keeping your chest up and knees out.

4. Drive up with the heels until fully extended.

5. Repeat.

Stiff-Leg Deadlift

Movement pattern: hinge | **Equipment:** none

1. Stand with your feet about hip-width apart, toes pointing forward, torso straight and knees slightly bent.

2. Keeping your knees stationary and your back straight, hinge at your hips and reach your hands down the front of your legs towards your toes. Keep moving forward as if you were going to pick something up from the floor until you feel a stretch on your hamstrings.

3. Squeeze your glutes, keep your back tight and drive your hips through to bring your torso up straight again to go back to the starting position.

4. Repeat.

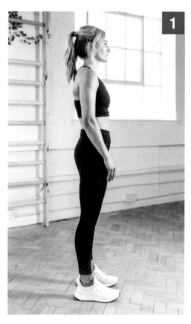

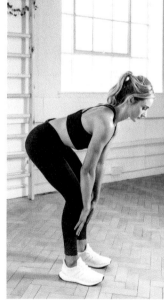

Split Squat

Movement pattern: lunge | **Equipment:** none

1. From a standing position, take a large step forwards as if performing a lunge. The heel of your back foot should be raised. Place your hands on your hips.

2. Keeping your torso straight, lower down slowly until your back knee almost touches the floor, then drive back up. Focus on keeping your knees in line with your toes, especially on the front leg, and ensure that the front knee does not stray past your toes as you lower.

3. Complete all your repetitions on one leg, then repeat with the other.

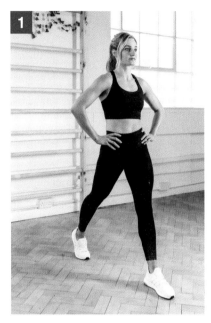
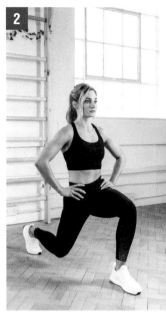

Glute Bridge

Movement pattern: hip extension | **Equipment:** none

1. Lie on your back with your knees bent at a 45-degree angle and your feet flat on the floor. Arms should be positioned down by your sides, with your palms down.

2. Push your lower back towards the floor to engage your core. Lift your hips off the ground until your knees, hips and shoulders form a straight line. Focus on pushing your knees away from your body, squeezing your glutes and lifting your hips up to the ceiling.

3. Hold your bridged position for a couple of seconds before easing back down towards the floor.

4. Repeat.

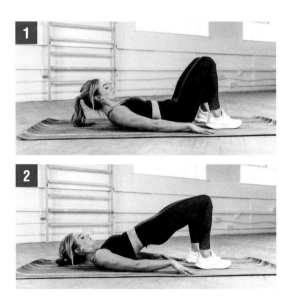

BEGINNER UPPER BODY EXERCISES

Press-Up

Movement pattern: push | **Equipment:** none

1. Start either on your knees or from an extended plank position with your hands underneath your shoulders.

2. Keep your body in a straight line from head to toe (or knees) without sagging in the middle or arching your back.

3. Engage your core by pulling your belly button towards your spine. Keep a tight core throughout the entire press-up.

4. Slowly bend your elbows, keeping them close to your body. Continue to lower yourself until your elbows are at approximately a 90-degree angle and your chest is close to the floor.

5. Push back up with your hands to the start position.

6. Repeat.

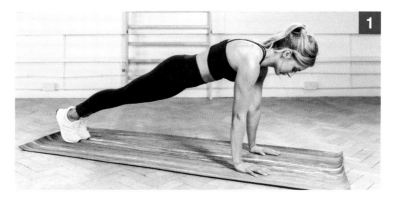

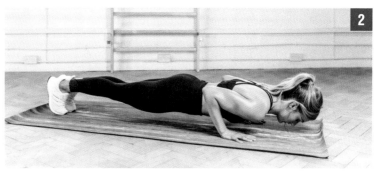

Prone Straight-Arm Raise

Movement pattern: pull | **Equipment:** none

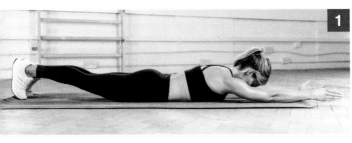

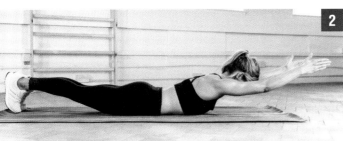

1. Lie face down on the floor with your arms stretched up above your head, thumbs up and palms facing one another. Your feet should be flexed with your toes on the floor. Keep your neck in a neutral position.

2. While continuing to look at the floor, tighten your core and keep your arms close to both sides of your head.

3. Slowly lift your arms off the floor towards the ceiling keeping them straight. Your upper chest should also be lifted a few inches off the floor. Hold for a few seconds.

4. Lower yourself back to the starting position.

5. Repeat.

Plank

Movement pattern: core | **Equipment:** none

1. Lie face down with your forearms on the floor and your elbows directly beneath your shoulders.

2. Keep your feet flexed with your toes on the floor.

3. Clasp your hands in front of your face, so your forearms make an inverted "V."

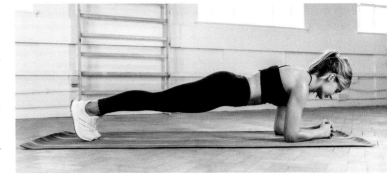

4. Rise up on your toes so that only your forearms and toes are touching the floor. Your body should hover a few inches off the floor in a straight line from your head to your feet.

5. Draw your bellybutton towards your spine to engage your core and squeeze your glutes. Look at the floor to keep your head in neutral position and breathe normally.

6. Hold the position for the recommended time or for 30-45 seconds.

Side Plank

Movement pattern: core | **Equipment:** none

1. Lie on one side with your elbow directly underneath your shoulder.

2. Extend your legs out straight and position your top foot either directly on top of your bottom foot or just in front of your bottom foot, whichever is more comfortable.

3. Engage your core and raise your hips until your body is in a straight line from your head to your feet. Your top arm can be stretched up above you to help you balance.

4. Hold the position for the recommended time, or for 30-45 seconds, without letting your hips drop.

5. Repeat on the opposite side.

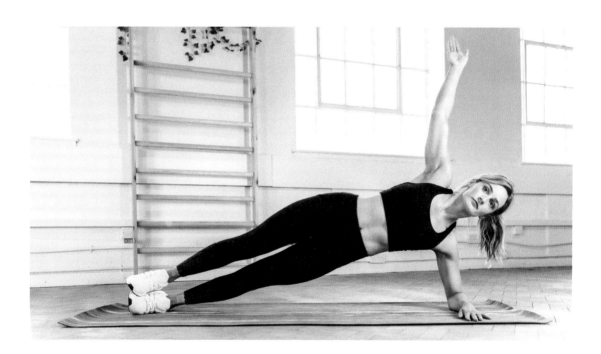

INTERMEDIATE LOWER BODY EXERCISES

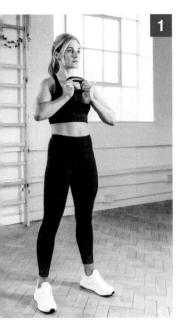

Goblet Squat

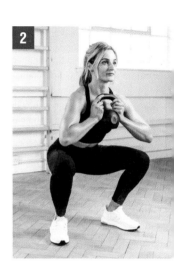

Movement pattern: squat | **Equipment:** kettlebell (or dumbbell)

1. Stand with your feet at shoulder-width apart and your toes pointed out slightly.

2. Hold the kettlebell at your chest.

3. Keep your chest up and engage your core, slowly squat down, ensuring that you continually drive your knees out, keeping them in line with your toes. Your weight should be back on your heels.

4. Drive back up until fully extended, keeping your chest up, knees out and squeezing your glutes.

5. Repeat.

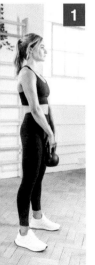
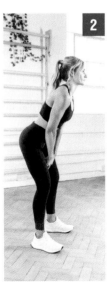
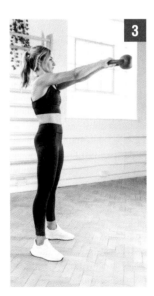

Kettlebell Swing

Movement pattern: hinge | **Equipment:** kettlebell

1. Hold the kettlebell handle with both hands.

2. Stand upright with your feet about shoulder-width apart.

3. Pull the kettlebell between your legs, sending your hips back with as little bend in your knees as possible. Keep your chest upright, pinching your shoulder blades together.

4. Drive your hips back through, using this force to drive the kettlebell up in front of you to eye level, keeping your arms straight.

5. Repeat.

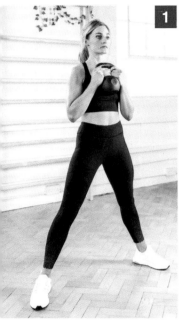
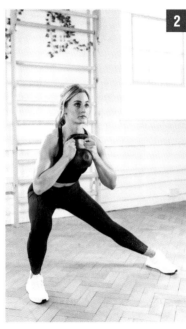

Lateral Lunge

Movement pattern: lunge | **Equipment:** kettlebell (or dumbbell or barbell)

1. Stand tall with your feet positioned in a wide stance and your toes pointing forward.

2. Hold the kettlebell at your chest.

3. Keeping your torso facing forwards and your weight back on your heels at all times, lower down to one side until the knee of your leading leg is bent to around 90 degrees. Keep your other leg straight. Always focus on bending and lowering from the hips, with your back straight and your core engaged.

4. Drive off the bent leg, pushing back up and returning to the starting position.

5. Repeat, leading with the opposite leg.

Hip Thrust

Movement pattern: hip extension | **Equipment:** dumbbell (or barbell) and bench/box

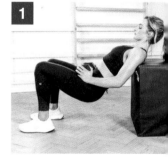

1. Begin in a seated position on the ground with the bench directly behind you.

2. Position so your shoulders and shoulder blades are on top of the bench (depending on the height of the bench or box, this may result in your hips coming off the floor slightly). Your feet should be hip-width apart and your knees should be bent at approximately 45° degrees in front of you with the soles of your feet on the floor. Your torso should be in a straight position, your body aligned and your spine neutral.

3. Hold each side of the dumbbell using both hands and place it at your hips.

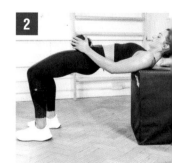

4. Drive through your heels and squeeze your glutes to lift your hips (and the dumbbell) vertically as high as possible. Your body weight should be supported by your shoulder blades and your feet. Tuck your chin towards your chest. Your tailbone should be tucked inwards, and your ribs should be pulled down. At the top, your shins should be vertical.

5. Come down smoothly, with your core still engaged to return to the starting position.

6. Repeat.

INTERMEDIATE UPPER BODY EXERCISES

Floor Press

Movement pattern: push | **Equipment:** dumbbells (or barbell)

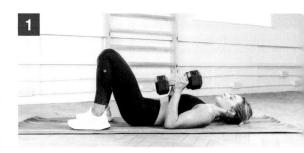

1. Lie with your back on the floor, your knees bent and your feet flat on the floor.

2. Holding a dumbbell in each hand, begin with your arms bent at approximately 90 degrees, with your upper arms in contact with the floor.

3. Drive the dumbbells towards the ceiling so the weights are fully extended above you, palms facing towards one another.

4. Pause at the top and then gradually return to the starting position, with your upper arms resting on the floor.

5. Repeat.

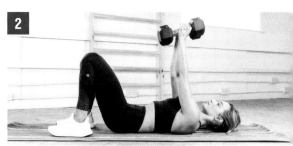

Renegade Row

Movement pattern: pull | **Equipment:** dumbbells

1. Holding a dumbbell in each hand, assume a plank position with straight arms. Your feet set slightly wider than shoulder-width apart.

2. Engage your core by pulling your belly button towards your spine. Pull one arm up into the body, keeping the elbow close and lifting the dumbbell off the floor towards your armpit.

3. Lower the dumbbell gently back to the floor to assume the starting position.

4. Repeat on the opposite side.

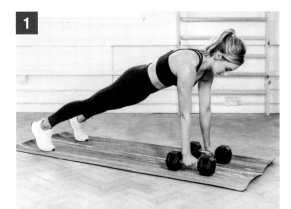

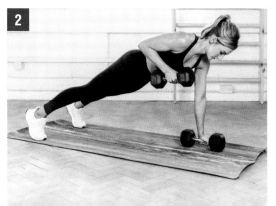

Pallof Press

Movement pattern: core | **Equipment:** resistance band

1. Loop a resistance band through itself on a squat rack (or another stable alternative) at chest height.

2. Stand sideways to the rack. Take the other end of the resistance band with both hands, one over the other, and hold it at your chest.

3. Take a step away from the rack, enough so the resistance band becomes taut. Stand with your feet shoulder-width apart, your knees slightly bent and your core engaged.

4. In an explosive movement, extend your arms and push the band away from you at chest height, until your arms reach full extension.

5. Keep your feet planted, your core engaged and your hips square as you hold this position for one to two seconds, then slowly return to the starting positon.

6. Repeat.

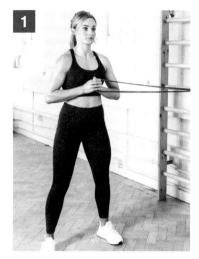
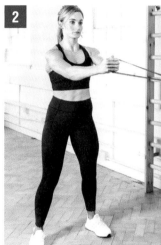

Mountain Climbers

Movement pattern: core | **Equipment:** none

1. Start in an extended plank position with your hands underneath your shoulders.

2. Bring one knee to your chest at a time, keeping your core engaged, your hips square and your weight over your hands.

3. Drive one knee to your chest at a time as fast as you can for the required time or for 30-45 seconds.

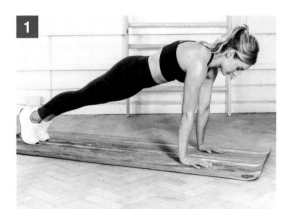
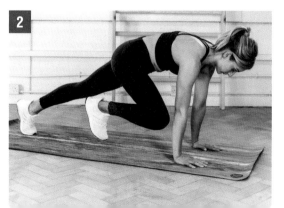

ADVANCED LOWER BODY EXERCISES

Overhead Squat

Movement pattern: squat | **Equipment:** kettlebells (or resistance band, dumbbells or barbell)

1. Stand with your feet shoulder-width apart and your toes turned out slightly.

2. With a kettlebell in each hand, hold them so they are resting on each shoulder with your hands next to your ears and your elbows pointing towards the floor.

3. Extend your arms up and push the kettlebells up above your head. Engage your core.

4. Slowly bend your knees, keeping your chest up and squat down until your thighs are parallel to the ground. Make sure your keep driving your knees out so they track in line with your toes. Your arms should remain straight with your hands shoulder-width apart. As you squat down, your arms should not track forward.

5. Drive up with your heels from the bottom of the squat, keeping your arms extended and the kettlebells above your head.

6. Repeat.

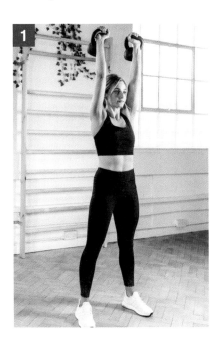
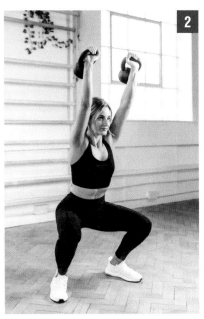

Single-Leg, Stiff-Leg Deadlift

Movement pattern: hinge | **Equipment:** kettlebell (or dumbbell or barbell)

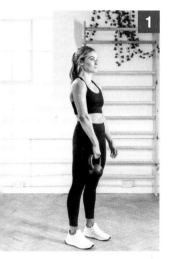
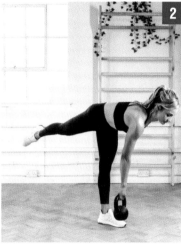

1. Hold the handle of a kettlebell in one hand.

2. Stand on the leg opposite the hand holding the kettlebell.

3. Keeping the knee of the standing leg slightly bent, begin to perform a stiff-leg deadlift by bending at the hip and extending your free leg behind you, aiming to get it parallel to the ground. Keep your shoulders back to maintain a neutral spine. Continue lowering the kettlebell towards the floor until your torso is parallel to the ground, or until you feel a stretch in your hamstrings.

4. Drive up through the standing leg, keeping your shoulders back, and return to the upright position.

5. Complete the number of repetitions on one leg before moving on to the other.

Bulgarian Split Squat

Movement pattern: lunge | **Equipment:** dumbbells (or kettlebells or barbell) and bench/box

1. Face away from the bench or box.

2. Hold a dumbbell in each hand down by your sides.

3. Place one foot behind you on top of the bench or box and assume the top of a lunge position.

4. Gently lower down into the bottom of a lunge position, ensuring that your front knee does not track over your toes.

5. Drive up until fully extended and repeat for the required number of repetitions.

6. Repeat on the opposite leg.

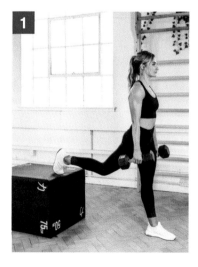
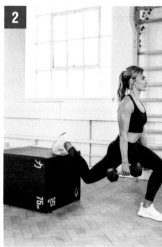

Feet-Elevated Glute Bridge

Movement pattern: hip extension | **Equipment:** dumbbell (or barbell) and bench/box

1. Place a bench (or box) parallel to the bottom of a mat.

2. Lie on the mat so your feet are closest to the bench.

3. Place both heels on top of the bench. Your feet should be hip-width apart.

4. Take your dumbbell and hold it in both hands at your hips.

5. Engage your core and drive your hips up towards the ceiling. Do this by driving through the heels and squeezing your glutes. Create a flat line with the body from your knees to your shoulders, making sure not to arch your lower back.

6. At the top position, hold for a second, then lower your hips back down until just off the floor.

7. Repeat.

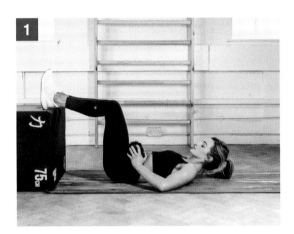
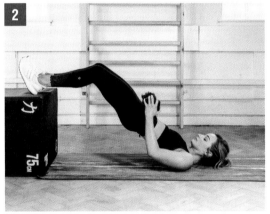

ADVANCED UPPER BODY EXERCISES

Pike Press-Up

Movement pattern: push | **Equipment:** none

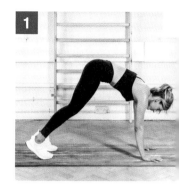

1. Assume an extended plank position on the floor. Your arms should be straight, and your hands should be underneath your shoulders.

2. Lift up your hips so that your body forms an upside-down V. Your legs and arms should stay as straight as possible, so you may need to adjust your feet until you feel comfortable.

3. Bend your elbows and lower your upper body until the top of your head nearly touches the floor.

4. Push yourself back up through your hands until your arms are straight.

5. Repeat.

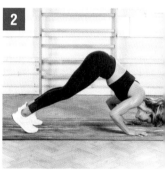

Bent-Over Row

Movement pattern: pull | **Equipment:** dumbbells (or resistance band, kettlebells or barbell)

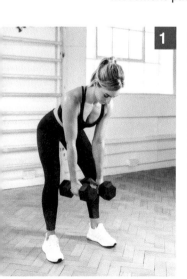
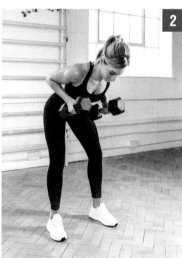

1. Stand with your feet hip-width apart.

2. Take a dumbbell in each hand, palms facing one another.

3. Keeping a flat, neutral spine, hinge from the hips, keeping your knees soft and slightly bent, and position the dumbbells just below your knees.

4. Pull the dumbbells up into the body, squeezing your shoulder blades together.

5. Lower the dumbbells gently back down to below your knees.

6. Repeat.

Side Plank Row

Movement pattern: core | **Equipment:** resistance band

1. Loop a resistance band round a squat rack (or other stable alternative) just higher than knee height.

2. Place a mat parallel with the squat rack, far enough away that the resistance band is taut when your arm is outstretched.

3. Lie on one side, facing the rack, with your elbow directly underneath your shoulder.

4. Have your legs out straight and position your top foot either directly on top of your bottom foot or just in front of your bottom foot, whichever is more comfortable.

5. Hold the loose end of the resistance band in your top hand (the hand not supporting your body weight). Remember, you should be far enough away that the resistance band is taut when your arm is outstretched.

6. Engage your core and raise your hips until your body is in a straight line from your head to your feet. Hold the position without letting your hips drop.

7. With the top arm extended, pull the resistance band towards the body, keeping your core engaged and elbow close to the body, all while avoiding any torso rotation.

8. Slowly extend your arm back to the outstretched starting position.

9. Complete the recommended number of repetitions on one arm before lowering yourself back to the floor. Position yourself on your opposite side to repeat using the other arm.

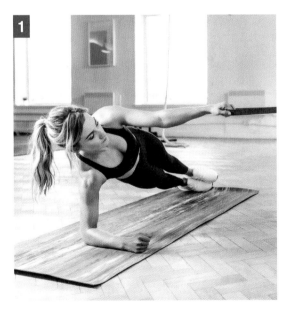
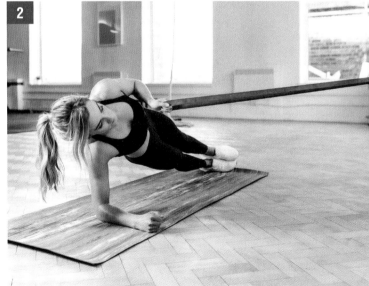

Dead Bug

Movement pattern: core | **Equipment:** kettlebell (or resistance band pulled taut around a rack)

1. Lie on your back on the floor.

2. Lift up your legs, bending your knees to 90 degrees and pointing your toes to the ceiling.

3. Hold the kettlebell in both hands and extend your arms directly above your chest.

4. Push your lower back into the floor, tucking your rib cage towards your hips.

5. Slowly drop one leg towards the floor, straightening it at the same time. Keep your toes pointing towards the ceiling and stop just before your leg touches the ground. Make sure you continue to push your lower back into the floor.

6. Bring your leg back to the starting position, next to your other knee. Repeat with the opposite leg, keeping your arms extended above your chest at all times.

7. Repeat.

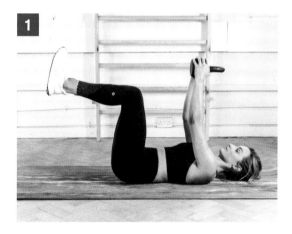
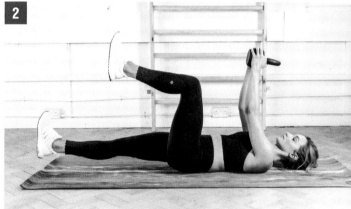

HIIT TRAINING METHODS

Tabata

Tabata is a type of HIIT which involves doing one exercise at high intensity for 20 seconds, followed by a 10 second rest, completing 8 rounds in total (i.e. 4 minutes of work). To apply this training method, you can focus on one exercise at a time, doing each for 4 minutes. This means if you complete a full-body workout, you should do the 8 exercises, working for 4 minutes on each one, giving you a 32-minute workout in total.

For example: 20 sec prisoner squats + 10 sec rest (x8) then move on to 20 sec straight-leg deadlifts + 10 sec rest (x8) and so on, to complete all your chosen exercises.

Personally, I like to mix Tabata up a little bit. I sometimes choose 2 lower-body exercises and 2 upper-body exercises to do together, rather than just focusing on one exercise at a time. For example: prisoner squat + straight-leg deadlift + press-ups + prone straight-arm raise.

The same 20:10 work-to-rest ratio still applies, meaning I would do each of these 4 exercises twice in the 4 minutes to complete 8 x 20 sec rounds.

How you decide to do it is entirely up to you. I also like to add Tabata-style 'finishers' to the end of my usual workouts at the gym, and maybe I'll just do one or two 4-minute rounds focusing on a few different exercises.

AMRAP

As Many Rounds/Reps As Possible. AMRAP is a form of HIIT whereby you try to complete as many rounds of a circuit (or repeats of an exercise) in a certain amount of time, taking as little rest as possible. The main aim is to focus on working at a high intensity and as hard as you can, but without compromising your exercise form. Doing AMRAPs can help you track your progress over time, as you can challenge yourself to complete more rounds in the same time frame the next time you do it.

To apply this training method, set the timer for anything between 10 and 30 minutes and perform 10 repetitions of each of your chosen exercises, as many times as possible within the set time. For example: Set your timer for 15 minutes and complete 10 repetitions of your chosen exercises repeatedly, until the timer stops.

For Time

A workout that's 'For Time' is a straight-forward workout where you do a certain number of repetitions of an exercise (or number of exercises) or rounds of an exercise circuit until you finish. The time when you complete all your repetitions or rounds is your score.

To apply this training method, choose your exercises and complete 10 repetitions of each one, completing between 3-5 rounds.

Example:

3 Rounds For Time of:

» 10 repetitions of prisoner squats

» 10 repetitions of stiff leg deadlift

» 10 repetitions of split squat

» Etc.

EMOM

Every Minute On the Minute.

An EMOM workout is a form of HIIT which involves doing a certain number of repetitions of an exercise, or number of exercises, every minute for a certain number of minutes. The quicker you complete the number of repetitions in each minute, the longer rest you will have before the next minute starts.

To apply this training method, choose between 1 and 3 exercises maximum, depending on your fitness level, and complete 10 repetitions of each exercise every minute for 10 minutes. Your aim is to exercise for roughly 45 seconds in each minute, so you have a short 10-15 second rest before the next minute starts, and you start again.

Example: Complete 10 x prisoner squats + 10 x straight-leg deadlifts every minute, for 10 minutes.

EMOMs are another training method that I prefer to use at the end of my usual workout at the gym, acting as a little high-intensity 'finisher' involving just a couple of exercises.

Ascending Ladder

An Ascending Ladder starts by completing one repetition of each of your chosen exercises, then increasing this by one additional repetition of each exercise, in the next round. This means the exercise gets harder each round as you add in more repetitions.

Example:

Round 1: 1 x prisoner squat, 1 x straight-leg deadlift, 1 x split squat, etc.

Round 2: 2 x prisoner squat, 2 x straight-leg deadlift, 2 x split squat, etc.

Continuing to increase the number of repetitions completed each round.

You have two options on how to complete this:

Example 1: You can set a time limit and try to complete as many rounds as possible in that time frame. I recommend a time limit of between 10-15 minutes.

OR

Example 2: You work up to a target number of repetitions of each exercise before stopping, taking a note of the time it took you to complete it. I recommend working your way up the ladder to reach a maximum of 10 repetitions of each exercise.

Descending Ladder

A Descending Ladder starts by completing a high number of repetitions of each exercise, then decreasing this by one less repetition of each exercise, in the next round. This means the workout starts hard but gets easier with each round as you decrease the number of repetitions you are completing.

Example:

Round 1: 10 x prisoner squat, 10 x straight-leg deadlift, 10 x split squat, etc.

Round 2: 9 x prisoner squat, 9 x straight-leg deadlift, 9 x split squat, etc.

Continuing to decrease the number of repetitions completed in each round until you reach zero.

I recommend starting with 10 repetitions of each of your chosen exercises and work your way down the ladder until you reach zero, taking a note of the time it took you to complete it.

Full Ladder

The Full Ladder incorporates both the Ascending and Descending Ladder and is a good one to complete if you have a little extra time!

To apply this training method, you begin with the ascending ladder, starting by completing 1 repetition of each exercise, increasing this number by an additional 1 repetition in each round, until you reach a target number of repetitions. Immediately after you have reached the target number of repetitions, you then begin the Descending Ladder and start to decrease the number of repetitions of each exercise you complete in each round.

Example:

Round 1: 1 x prisoner squat, 1 x straight-leg deadlift, 1 x split squat, etc.

Round 2: 2 x prisoner squat, 2 x straight-leg deadlift, 2 x split squat, etc.

...

Round 10: 10 x prisoner squat, 10 x straight-leg deadlift, 10 x split squat, etc.

Round 11: 9 x prisoner squat, 9 x straight-leg deadlift, 9 x split squat, etc.

Round 12: 8 x prisoner squat, 8 x straight-leg deadlift, 8 x split squat, etc.

Continue to decrease the number of repetitions until you reach zero, taking a note of the time it took you to complete it.

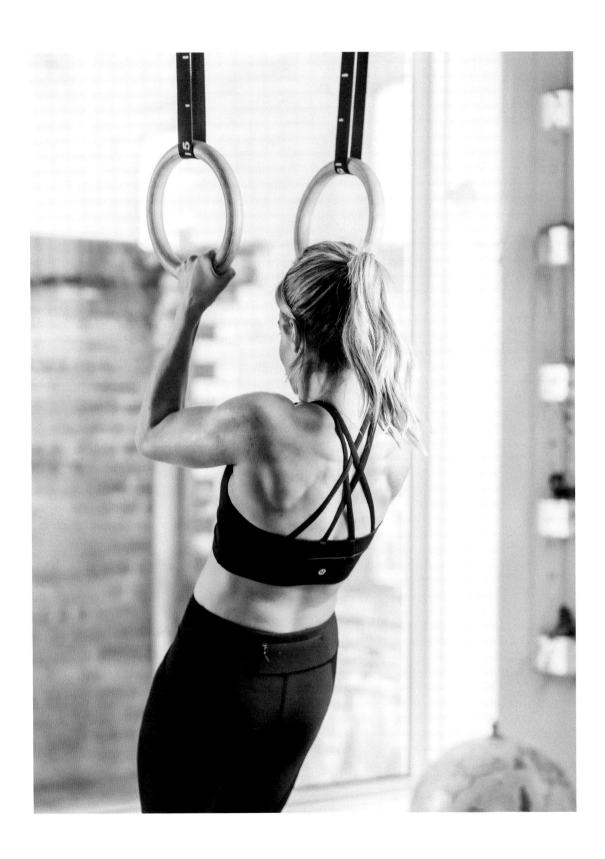

Start Your Journey to Nourishment

I really hope you have found the information in this book to be both interesting and informative. It is one of my biggest passions to help others understand the basics of nutrition, so that everyone has the power to make educated and informed food choices to help them lead healthy and happy lives.

I hope this book will help you to identify and avoid the nutrition nonsense being published on the internet and in some "health and fitness" magazines and guide you on a far more enjoyable and rewarding path to health. I will continue to shout loud and clear about being more mindful of where, and more importantly, who you get your health and nutrition information from. I can't stress enough that if you feel you need additional support with any aspect of your health or well-being, that you please go and speak to a qualified health professional.

I really hope you learn to fall in love with looking after yourself and that you now feel empowered to start your journey towards a healthier, happier and more fulfilling life. I really do hope that by reading this book you will also believe in my philosophy that nutrition and exercise can be simple, affordable and most importantly for you, enjoyable.

Don't forget to follow me on Instagram! @the_dietitian_kitchen

I would love to hear from you and hear your thoughts on the book.

References

CARBOHYDRATES

BRITISH DIETETIC ASSOCIATION (BDA) 2016. *Food Fact Sheet – Carbohydrates* [online] [Viewed 29 January 2019]. Available from: https://www.bda.uk.com/foodfacts/Carbs.pdf

BRITISH DIETETIC ASSOCIATION (BDA) 2016. *Food Fact Sheet – Fibre* [online] [Viewed 14 February 2019]. Available from: https://www.bda.uk.com/foodfacts/fibre_fact_sheet_poster

DIABETES UK. *Glycaemic Index and Diabetes* [online] [Viewed 12 February 2019]. Available from: https://www.diabetes.org.uk/guide-to-diabetes/enjoy-food/carbohydrates-and-diabetes/glycaemic-index-and-diabetes?gclid=EAIaIQobChMItPapm8624AIVjZXtCh2IVgRdEAAYASAAEgKPrPD_BwE

DIABETES UK. *What is Type 1 Diabetes?* [online] [Viewed 12 February 2019]. Available from: https://www.diabetes.org.uk/diabetes-the-basics/what-is-type-1-diabetes

DIABETES UK. *What is Type 2 Diabetes?* [online] [Viewed 12 February 2019]. Available from: https://www.diabetes.org.uk/diabetes-the-basics/what-is-type-2-diabetes

DIABETES UK. *Diabetes Risk Factors* [online] [Viewed 12 February 2019]. Available from: https://www.diabetes.org.uk/preventing-type-2-diabetes/diabetes-risk-factors

DIABETES UK. *Preventing Type 2 Diabetes*. [online] [Viewed 12 February 2019]. Available from: https://www.diabetes.org.uk/preventing-type-2-diabetes

DIABETES UK. *How can I reduce my risk of Type 2 Diabetes?* [online] [Viewed 12 February 2019]. Available from: https://www.diabetes.org.uk/preventing-type-2-diabetes/can-diabetes-be-prevented

MERGENTHALER, P., LINDAUER, U., DIENEL, G., MEISEL, A., 2013. Sugar for the brain: the role of glucose in physiological and pathological brain function. *Trends Neurosci*. October, vol. 36, no. 10, pp. 587-597.

NHS 2018. *Eat well; How to get more fibre into your diet*. [online] [Viewed 14 February 2019]. Available from: https://www.nhs.uk/live-well/eat-well/how-to-get-more-fibre-into-your-diet/

NHS 2018. *Eat well; Water, drinks and your health*. [online] [Viewed 14 February 2019]. Available from: https://www.nhs.uk/live-well/eat-well/water-drinks-nutrition/

NHS, 2018. *What is the glycaemic index (GI)?* [online] [Viewed 29 January 2019]. Available from: https://www.nhs.uk/common-health-questions/food-and-diet/what-is-the-glycaemic-index-gi/

SCIENTIFIC ADVISORY COMMITTEE ON NUTRITION (SACN), 2015. *SACN Carbohydrates and Health Report* [online] [Viewed 29 January 2019]. Available from: https://www.gov.uk/government/publications/sacn-carbohydrates-and-health-report

PROTEIN

BRITISH DIETETIC ASSOCIATION (BDA) 2014. *Vegetarian Diets*. [online] [Viewed 14 February 2019]. Available at: https://www.bda.uk.com/foodfacts/vegetarianfoodfacts.pdf

BRITISH NUTRITION FOUNDATION (BNF) 2017. *Healthy eating for vegans and vegetarians*. [online] [Viewed 14 February 2019]. Available at: https://www.nutrition.org.uk/healthyliving/helpingyoueatwell/veganandvegetarian.html?limit=1&start=11

BRITISH NUTRITION FOUNDATION (BNF) 2016. *Nutrition Requirements*. [online] [Viewed 14 February 2019]. Available at: https://www.nutrition.org.uk/attachments/article/234/Nutrition%20Requirements_Revised%20Oct%202016.pdf

BRITISH NUTRITION FOUNDATION (BNF) 2012. *Protein*. [online] [Viewed February 14 2019]. Available from: https://www.nutrition.org.uk/nutritionscience/nutrients-food-and-ingredients/protein.html

AMERICAN COLLEGE OF SPORTS MEDICINE (ACSM), 2015. *Protein Intake for Optimal Muscle Maintenance*. [online] [Viewed February 14 2019]. Available from: https://www.acsm.org/docs/default-source/files-for-resource-library/protein-intake-for-optimal-muscle-maintenance.pdf

WESTERTERP, K.R. 2004. Diet induced thermogenesis. *Nutrition & Metabolism*. August, vol. 1, no. 5.

FAT

BRITISH DIETETIC ASSOCIATION (BDA), 2018. *Food Fact Sheet: Fats*. [online] [Viewed 15 February 2019]. Available from: https://www.bda.uk.com/foodfacts/FatFacts.pdf

BRITISH DIETETIC ASSOCIATION (BDA), 2017. *Food Fact Sheet: Omega-3*. [online] [Viewed 16 February 2019]. Available from: https://www.bda.uk.com/foodfacts/omega3.pdf

BRITISH NUTRITION FOUNDATION (BNF), 2012. *Fat*. [online] [Viewed 15 February 2019]. Available from: https://www.nutrition.org.uk/nutritionscience/nutrients-food-and-ingredients/fat.html

BRITISH NUTRITION FOUNDATION (BNF), 2017. *Good fats and bad fats explained*. [online] [Viewed 15 February 2019]. Available from: https://www.nutrition.org.uk/healthyliving/helpingyoueatwell/fats.html

BRITISH NUTRITION FOUNDATION (BNF), 2017. *Heart Disease*. [online] [Viewed 15 February 2019]. Available from: https://www.nutrition.org.uk/nutritionscience/health-conditions/heart-disease.html

NHS, 2018. *Healthy Body: Lower Your Cholesterol*. [online] [Viewed 16 February 2019]. Available from: https://www.nhs.uk/live-well/healthy-body/lower-your-cholesterol/

NHS, 2018. *High Cholesterol: Causes*. [online] [Viewed 16 February 2019]. Available from: https://www.nhs.uk/conditions/high-cholesterol/causes/

NHS, 2017. *Eat well; Fat: The Facts*. [online] [Viewed 15 February 2019]. Available from: https://www.nhs.uk/live-well/eat-well/different-fats-nutrition/#trans-fats

QIAN, F., KORAT, A.A., MALIK, V. and HU, F.B., 2016. Metabolic Effects of Monounsaturated Fatty Acid-Enriched Diets Compared With Carbohydrate or Polyunsaturated Fatty Acid-Enriched Diets in Patients With Type 2 Diabetes: A Systematic Review and Meta-analysis of Randomized Controlled Trials. *Diabetes Care*. August, vol. 39, no. 8, pp. 1448-1457.

SIMOPOULOS, A.P., 2006. Evolutionary aspects of diet, the omega-6/omega-3 ratio and genetic variation: nutritional implications for chronic diseases. *Biomedicine and Pharmacotherapy*. November, vol. 60, no. 9, pp. 502-507.

CALORIES

BRITISH DIETETIC ASSOCIATION (BDA), 2016. *Food Fact Sheet: Energy Density*. [online] [Viewed 16 February 2019]. Available from: https://www.bda.uk.com/foodfacts/energydensityfoodfactsheet

BRITISH NUTRITION FOUNDATION (BNF), 2009. *Energy intake and expenditure*. [online] [Viewed 16 February 2019]. Available from: https://www.nutrition.org.uk/nutritionscience/obesityandweightmanagement/energy-intake-and-expenditure.html

BRITISH NUTRITION FOUNDATION (BNF), 2018. *The Quality Calorie (QC) Concept*. [online] [Viewed 16 February 2019]. Available from: https://www.nutrition.org.uk/healthyliving/helpingyoueatwell/qualitycalorie.html

WESTERTERP, K.R. 2004. Diet induced thermogenesis. *Nutrition & Metabolism*. August, vol. 1, no. 5.

WESTERTERP, K.R., WILSON, S.A.J. and ROLLAND, V., 1999. Diet induced thermogenesis measured over 24h in a respiration chamber: effect of diet composition. *International Journal of Obesity*. February, vol. 23, pp. 287-292.

MICRONUTRIENTS

BRITISH NUTRITION FOUNDATION (BNF), 2016. *Exploring Nutrients*. [online] [Viewed 16 February 2019]. Available from: https://www.nutrition.org.uk/healthyliving/basics/exploring-nutrients.html

NHS, 2017. *Vitamins and Minerals*. [online] [Viewed 16 February 2019]. Available from https://www.nhs.uk/conditions/vitamins -and-minerals/others/

THOMAS, B. and BISHOP, J., 2007. *Manual of Dietetic Practice*, (Fourth Edition), Kent: Blackwell.

SALT

BRITISH DIETETIC ASSOCIATION (BDA), 2016. *Food Fact Sheet: Salt and Health*. [online] [Viewed 16 February 2019]. Available from: https://www.bda.uk.com/foodfacts/Salt.pdf

BRITISH HEART FOUNDATION (BHF), 2015. [online] [Viewed 16 February 2019]. Available from: https://www.bhf.org.uk/informationsupport/risk-factors/high-blood-pressure

BRITISH NUTRITION FOUNDATION (BNF), 2009. *Minerals and trace elements: Sodium*. [online] [Viewed 16 February 2019]. Available from: https://www.nutrition.org.uk/nutritionscience/nutrients-food-and-ingredients/minerals-and-trace-elements.html?start=6

NHS, 2018. *Eat Well: Salt – The Facts*. [online] [Viewed 16 February 2019]. Available from: https://www.nhs.uk/live-well/eat-well/salt-nutrition/#salt-or-sodium

THOMAS, B. and BISHOP, J., 2007. *Manual of Dietetic Practice*, (Fourth Edition), Kent: Blackwell.

BONE HEALTH

BRITISH DIETETIC ASSOCIATION (BDA), 2017. *Food Fact Sheet: Calcium*. [online] [Viewed 17 February 2019]. Available from: https://www.bda.uk.com/foodfacts/Calcium.pdf

BRITISH DIETETIC ASSOCIATION (BDA), 2016. *Food Fact Sheet: Vitamin D*. [online] [Viewed 17 February 2019]. Available from: https://www.bda.uk.com/foodfacts/VitaminD.pdf

BRITISH DIETETIC ASSOCIATION (BDA), 2016. *Food Fact Sheet: Osteoporosis*. [online] [Viewed 17 February 2019]. Available from: https://www.bda.uk.com/foodfacts/osteoporosis.pdf

BRITISH NUTRITION FOUNDATION (BNF), 2018. *Bone and joint health*. [online] [Viewed 17 February 2019]. Available from: https://www.nutrition.org.uk/nutritionscience/health-conditions/bone-and-joint-health.html

BRITISH NUTRITION FOUNDATION (BNF), 2016. *New reports: New advice on Vitamin D*. [online] [Viewed 17 February 2019]. Available from: https://www.nutrition.org.uk/nutritioninthenews/new-reports/983-newvitamind.html

BRITISH NUTRITION FOUNDATION (BNF), 2015. *Factsheet: Nutrition, health and schoolchildren: Bone health*. [online] [Viewed 17 February 2019]. Available from: https://www.nutrition.org.uk/attachments/article/546/Nutrition,%20health%20and%20schoolchildren_Bone%20health%20factsheet_updated.pdf

INTERNATIONAL OSTEOPORSIS FOUNDATION, 2015. *A bone-healthy lifestyle in the teenage years pays off*. [online] [Viewed 17 February 2019]. Available from: https://www.iofbonehealth.org/news/bone-healthy-lifestyle-teenage-years-pays

NHS, 2016. *Conditions: Osteoporosis*. [online] [Viewed 17 February 2019]. Available from: https://www.nhs.uk/conditions/osteoporosis/

NHS, 2017. *Conditions: Vitamins & Minerals; Vitamin D*. [online] [Viewed 17 February 2019]. Available from: https://www.nhs.uk/conditions/vitamins-and-minerals/vitamin-d/

PITUKCHEEWANONT, P., AUSTIN, J., CHEN, P. and PUNYASAVATSUT, N., 2013. Bone health in children and adolescents: risk factors for low bone density. *Paediatric Endocrinology Reviews*. March, vol. 10, no. 3, pp. 318-335.

THOMAS, B. and BISHOP, J., 2007. *Manual of Dietetic Practice*, (Fourth Edition), Kent: Blackwell.

WEAVER, C.M., GORDON, C.M., JANZ, K.F., KALKWARF, H.J., LAPPE, J.M., LEWIS, R., O'KARMA, M., WALLACE, T.C. and ZEMEL, B.S., 2016. The National Osteoporosis Foundation's position statement on peak bone mass development and lifestyle factors: a systematic review and implementation recommendations. *Osteoporosis International*. April, vol. 27, no. 4, pp. 1281-1386.

HYDRATION

BRITISH DIETETIC ASSOCIATION (BDA), 2017. *Food Fact Sheet: Fluid*. [online] [Viewed 17 February 2019]. Available from: https://www.bda.uk.com/foodfacts/fluid.pdf

BRITISH NUTRITION FOUNDATION (BNF), 2018. *Healthy Hydration Guide*. [online] [Viewed 17 February 2019]. Available from: https://www.nutrition.org.uk/healthyliving/hydration/healthy-hydration-guide.html

THOMAS, B. and BISHOP, J., 2007. *Manual of Dietetic Practice*, (Fourth Edition), Kent: Blackwell.

BUILDING A BALANCED PLATE

BRITISH DIETETIC ASSOCIATION (BDA), 2016. *Food Fact Sheet: Healthy Eating*. [online] [Viewed 18 February 2019]. Available from: https://www.bda.uk.com/foodfacts/HealthyEating.pdf

BRITISH NUTRITION FOUNDATION (BNF), 2019. *Find your balance – get portion wise!* [online] [Viewed 18 February 2019]. Available from: https://www.nutrition.org.uk/healthyliving/find-your-balance/portionwise.html

FOOD LABELLING

BRITISH DIETETIC ASSOCIATION (BDA), 2018. *Food Fact Sheet. Food Labelling: Nutrition Information*. [online] [Viewed 18 February 2019]. Available from: https://www.bda.uk.com/foodfacts/labelling.pdf

BRITISH NUTRITION FOUNDATION (BNF), 2016. *Helping you eat well. Looking at Labels: Front of pack labelling*. [online] [Viewed 18 February 2019]. Available from: https://www.nutrition.org.uk/healthyliving/helpingyoueatwell/324-labels.html?start=3

BUSTING NUTRITION MYTHS

BRITISH DIETETIC ASSOCIATION (BDA), 2016. *Food Fact Sheet: Detox Diets*. [online] [Viewed 19 February 2019]. Available from: https://www.bda.uk.com/foodfacts/detoxdiets.pdf

BRITISH DIETETIC ASSOCIATION (BDA), 2017. *Top 5 worst celeb diets to avoid in 2018*. [Viewed 19 February 2019]. Available from: https://www.bda.uk.com/news/view?id=195

BRITISH NUTRITION FOUNDATION (BNF), 2018. *FAQs: Cancer – Nutrition Myths.* [online] [Viewed 19 February 2019]. Available from: https://www.nutrition.org.uk/attachments/article/1158/BNF%20 FAQs%20cancer%20and%20nutrition%20myths_final_V3.pdf

BRITISH NUTRITION FOUNDTION (BNF), 2009. *Lactose Intolerance.* [online] [Viewed 19 February 2019]. Available from: https://www.nutrition.org.uk/nutritionscience/allergy/lactose-intolerance.html

BRITISH NUTRITION FOUNDATION (BNF), 2009. *Wheat intolerance and coeliac disease.* [online] [Viewed 19 February 2019]. Available from: https://www.nutrition.org.uk/nutritionscience/allergy/wheat-intolerance-and-coeliac-disease.html

CHEST, HEART AND STROKE SCOTLAND, 2016. *Superfood or Super-fad: Is there truth to the health claims?* [online] [Viewed 19 February 2019]. Available from: https://www.chss.org.uk/supportus/hps/superfood-or-super-fad/

COELIAC UK, no date. *Coeliac Disease.* [online] [Viewed 19 February 2019]. Available from: https://www.coeliac.org.uk/coeliac-disease/

NHS CHOICES, 2011. *Miracle Foods: Myths and The Media.* [online] [Viewed 19 February 2019]. Available from: https://www.nhs.uk/news/2011/02February/Documents/BTH_Miracle_%20foods_report.pdf

THE DAIRY COUNCIL, 2016. *Milk: Fact Sheet.* [online] [Viewed 19 February 2019]. Available from: https://www.milk.co.uk/hcp/wp-content/uploads/sites/2/woocommerce_uploads/2016/12/Milk_consumer_2016.pdf

FOOD & GUT HEALTH

BRITISH DIETETIC ASSOCIATION (BDA), 2016. *Food Fact Sheet: Irritable Bowel Syndrome and Diet.* [online] [Viewed 19 February 2019]. Available from: https://www.bda.uk.com/foodfacts/IBSfoodfacts.pdf

BRITISH DIETETIC ASSOCIATION (BDA), 2018. *Food Fact Sheet: Probiotics.* [online] [Viewed 19 February 2019]. Available from: https://www.bda.uk.com/foodfacts/probiotics.pdf

BRITISH NUTRITION FOUNDATION (BNF), 2016. *Functional Foods.* [online] [Viewed 19 February 2019]. Available from: https://www.nutrition.org.uk/nutritionscience/foodfacts/functional-foods.html

NATIONAL INSTITUTE FOR HEALTH AND CARE EXCELLENCE (NICE), 2015. *Irritable Bowel Syndrome.* [online] [Viewed 20 February 2019]. Available from: https://bnf.nice.org.uk/treatment-summary/irritable-bowel-syndrome.html

NHS, 2017. *Diet, lifestyle and medicines: Irritable Bowel Syndrome (IBS).* [online] [Viewed 19 February 2019]. Available from: https://www.nhs.uk/conditions/irritable-bowel-syndrome-ibs/diet-lifestyle-and-medicines/

NHS, 2016. *Eat well: Good foods to help your digestion.* [online] [Viewed 19 February 2019]. Available from: https://www.nhs.uk/live-well/eat-well/good-foods-to-help-your-digestion/#cut-down-on-fat-for-a-healthy-gut

THOMAS, B. and BISHOP, J., 2007. *Manual of Dietetic Practice*, (Fourth Edition), Kent: Blackwell.

FOOD & MOOD

BRITISH DIETETIC ASSOCIATION (BDA), 2017. *Food Fact Sheet: Food and Mood*. [online] [Viewed 20 February 2018]. Available from: https://www.bda.uk.com/foodfacts/foodmood.pdf

BRITISH DIETETIC ASSOCIATION (BDA), 2017. *Food Fact Sheet: Omega-3*. [online] [Viewed 20 February 2019]. Available from: https://www.bda.uk.com/foodfacts/omega3.pdf

FOOD & SKIN HEALTH

BRITISH DIETETIC ASSOCIATION (BDA), 2016. *Food Fact Sheet: Skin health*. [online] [Viewed 20 February 2019]. Available from: https://www.bda.uk.com/foodfacts/SkinHealth.pdf

BRITISH NUTRITION FOUNDATION (BNF), 2018. *Five Fast Facts on Nutrition and Skin*. [online] [Viewed 20 February 2019]. Available from: https://www.nutrition.org.uk/attachments/article/1126/BNF%20Five%20Fast%20Facts%20on%20Nutrition%20and%20Skin.pdf

NHS, 2016. *Conditions: Acne*. [online] [Viewed 20 February 2019]. Available from: https://www.nhs.uk/conditions/acne/

PLANT-BASED DIETS

BRITISH DIETETIC ASSOCIATION (BDA), 2016. *Food Fact Sheet: Iodine*. [online] [Viewed 21 February 2019]. Available from: https://www.bda.uk.com/foodfacts/Iodine.pdf

BRITISH DIETETIC ASSOCIATION (BDA), 2017. *Food Fact Sheet: Plant-based diet*. [online] [Viewed 21 February 2019]. Available from: https://www.bda.uk.com/foodfacts/plantbaseddiets.pdf

WILLETT, W., ROCKSTRÖM, J., LOKEN, B., SPRINGMANN, M., LANG, T., VERMEULEN, S., 2019. Food in the Anthropocene: the EAT−Lancet Commission on healthy diets from sustainable food systems. *The Lancet Commissions*. Vol. 393, no. 10170, pp. 447-492.

IMPROVING YOUR RELATIONSHIP WITH FOOD

BEAT EATING DISORDERS, 2016. *Emotional Overeating*. [online] [Viewed 21 February 2019]. Available from: https://www.beateatingdisorders.org.uk/types/emotional-overeating

BURGGRAF, F. and MEGRETTE, F., 2010. *Discover Mindful Eating: A Resource of Handouts for Health Professionals*. Arlington, Virginia: Skelly.

DAUBENMIER, J., MORAN, P.J., KRISTELLER, J., ACREE, M., BACCHETTI, P., KEMENY, M.E., DALLMAN, M., LUSTIG, R.H., GRUNFELD, C., NIXON, D.F., MILUSH, J.M., GOLDMAN, V., LARAIA, B., LAUGERO, K.D., WOODHOUSE, L., EPEL, E.S. and HECHT, F.M., 2016. Effects of a Mindfulness-Based Weight Loss Intervention in Adults with Obesity: A Randomized Clinical Trial. *Obesity*. Vol. 24, no. 4, pp. 794-804.

FLETCHER, M., 2017. *The Core Concepts in Mindful Eating: Professional Edition*. Epping: Self-publisher.

KIDD, L.I., GRAOR, C.H. and MURROCK, C.J., 2013. A mindful eating group intervention for obese women: a mixed methods feasibility study. *Archives of Psychiatric Nursing*. Vol. 27, pp. 211-218.

MATHIEU, J., 2009. Topics of Professional Interest. What should you know about mindful and intuitive eating? *Journal of the Academy of Nutrition and Dietetics*. Vol. 109, no. 12, pp. 1982-1987.

O'REILLY, G. A., COOK, L., SPRUIJT-METZ, D. and BLACK, D.S., 2014. Mindfulness-based interventions for obesity-related eating behaviours: a literature review. *International Association for the Study of Obesity*. Vol. 15, pp. 453-461.

BEING YOUR OWN MOTIVATION

THOMAS, B. and BISHOP, J., 2007. *Manual of Dietetic Practice*, (Fourth Edition), Kent: Blackwell.

SLEEP

NATIONAL SLEEP FOUNDATION, 2018. *Healthy Sleep Tips*. [online] [Viewed 22 February 2019]. Available from: https://www.sleepfoundation.org/articles/healthy-sleep-tips

NHS, 2016. *Sleep and tiredness*. [online] [Viewed 22 February 2019]. Available from: https://www.nhs.uk/live-well/sleep-and-tiredness/how-to-get-to-sleep/?tabname=sleep-tips

ALCOHOL

BRITISH DIETETIC ASSOCIATION (BDA), 2016. *Food Fact Sheet: Alcohol*. [online] [Viewed 22 February 2019]. Available from: https://www.bda.uk.com/foodfacts/Alcohol.pdf

NHS, 2018. *Alcohol Support: Alcohol Units*. [online] [Viewed 22 February 2019]. Available from: https://www.nhs.uk/live-well/alcohol-support/calculating-alcohol-units/

GETTING ACTIVE

NHS, 2018. *Exercise: Physical Activity Guidelines for Adults*. [online] [Viewed 23 February 2019]. Available from: https://www.nhs.uk/live-well/exercise/

NHS, 2018. *Exercise: Benefits of Exercise*. [online] [Viewed 23 February 2019]. Available from: https://www.nhs.uk/live-well/exercise/exercise-health-benefits/

NUTRITION FOR FITNESS

AMERICAN COLLEGE OF SPORTS MEDICINE, 2007. Exercise and Fluid Replacement. *Medicine and Science in Sports & Exercise*. February, vol. 39, no. 2, pp. 377-390.

AMERICAN COLLEGE OF SPORTS MEDICINE, 2016. Nutrition and Athletic Performance: Joint Position Statement. *Medicine and Science in Sports & Exercise*. March, vol. 48, no.3, pp. 543-568.

BRITISH DIETETIC ASSOCIATION (BDA), 2017. *Food Fact Sheet: Sport*. [online] [Viewed 23 February 2019]. Available from: https://www.bda.uk.com/foodfacts/sportsfoodfacts.pdf

INTERNATIONAL OLYMPIC COMMITTEE (IOC), 2018. IOC Consensus Statement: Dietary Supplements and the High-Performance Athlete. *International Journal of Sport Nutrition and Exercise Metabolism*. April, vol. 28, pp. 104-125.

Recipe Index

Sweet Indulgence

Dips & Spreads

Exercise Index

Conversion Charts

Dry Weights

Metric	Imperial
5g	1/4 oz
8/10g	1/3 oz
15g	1/2 oz
20g	3/4 oz
25g	1oz
30/35g	1 1/4 oz
40g	1 1/2 oz
50g	2 oz
60/70g	2 1/2 oz
75/85/90g	3 oz
100g	3 1/2 oz
110/120g	4 oz
125/130g	4 1/2 oz
135/140/150g	5oz
170/175g	6oz
200g	7oz
225g	8oz
250g	9oz
265g	9 1/2 oz
275g	10oz
300g	11oz
325g	11 1/2 oz
350g	12oz

375g	13oz
400g	14oz
425g	15oz
450g	1lb
475g	1lb 1oz
500g	1lb 2oz
550g	1lb 3oz
600g	1lb 5oz
625g	1lb 6oz
650g	1lb 7oz
675g	1 1/2 lb
700g	1lb 9oz
750g	1lb 10oz
800g	1 3/4 lb
850g	1lb 14oz
900g	2lb
950g	2lb 2oz
1kg	2lb 3oz

Liquid Measures

Metric	Imperial	Cups
15ml	1/2 fl oz	1 tbsp (level)
20ml	3/4 fl oz	
25ml	1 fl oz	1/8 cup
30ml	1 1/4 fl oz	
50ml	2 fl oz	1/4 cup
60ml	2 1/2 fl oz	
75ml	3 fl oz	
100ml	3 1/2 fl oz	3/8 cup
110/120ml	4 fl oz	1/2 cup
125ml	4 1/2 fl oz	
150ml	5 fl oz	2/3 cup
175ml	6 fl oz	3/4 cup
200/215ml	7 fl oz	
225ml	8 fl oz	1 cup
250ml	9 fl oz	
275ml	9 1/2 fl oz	
300ml	1/2 pint	1 1/4 cups
350ml	12 fl oz	1 1/2 cups
375ml	13 fl oz	
400ml	14 fl oz	
425ml	15 fl oz	
450ml	16 fl oz	2 cups
500ml	18 fl oz	2 1/4 cups
550ml	19 fl oz	
600ml	1 pint	2 1/2 cups
700ml	1 1/4 pints	

750ml	1 1/3 pints	
800ml	1 pint, 9 fl oz	
850ml	1 1/2 pints	
900ml	1 pint, 12 fl oz	3 3/4 cups
1 litre	1 3/4 pints	4 cups

Oven Temperatures*

°C	°F	Gas Mark
110	225	1/4
130	250	1/2
140	275	1
150	300	2
160/170	325	3
180	350	4
190	375	5
200	400	6
220	425	7
230	450	8
240	475	9

*The temperatures indicated in the recipes are all based on using a fan-assisted oven. If you are using a conventional oven, increase the temperature by 20°C.

About the Author

Kerri achieved a first-class honours degree in Human Nutrition and Dietetics in 2012 and gained her Postgraduate Certificate (with Merit) in Sports Nutrition in 2015. She is a Registered Dietitian and graduate member of the Sports and Exercise Nutrition Register (SENr) in the United Kingdom. She currently works within the National Health Service (NHS), specialising in Surgical & Critical Care but also covers Gastroenterology, Respiratory, Cardiology, Orthopaedics, Rehabilitation, Stroke and General Medicine. Over and above her NHS job, Kerri also specialises in Sports Nutrition and does freelance work, supporting athletic individuals and sports teams on how to optimise their nutritional intake to enhance their performance. She also runs fitness classes and is a personal trainer in her local area, encouraging and motivating people to find their love of being active.

Credits

Cover & interior design: Annika Naas

Layout: Guido Maetzing, www.mmedia-agentur.de

Cover & interior photos: © Daniel McAvoy, www.danielmcavoy.co.uk

Managing editor: Elizabeth Evans

Copyeditor: Gloria J. Matzig